Introduction to Speech Science

From Basic Theories to Clinical Applications

Jack Ryalls
University of Central Florida

Susan Behrens
Marymount Manhattan College

Allyn and Bacon

Boston • London • Toronto • Sydney • Tokyo • Singapore

To mornings in Margate, and especially to Tony. SJB
To WAP and 'La Dolce Vita.' JR

Executive Editor: *Stephen D. Dragin*
Editorial Assistant: *Bridget McSweeney*
Senior Editorial-Production Administrator: *Joe Sweeney*
Editorial-Production Service: *Walsh & Associates, Inc.*
Composition Buyer: *Linda Cox*
Manufacturing Buyer: *Dave Repetto*
Cover Administrator: *Jenny Hart*

Library of Congress Cataloging-in-Publication Data

Ryalls, Jack H., 1954–
    Introduction to speech science : from basic theories to clinical
applications / Jack Ryalls, Susan Behrens.
        p.   cm.
    Includes bibliographical references and index.
    ISBN 0-205-29100-7
    1. Speech therapy.   2. Speech disorders.   3. Speech.   I. Behrens,
Susan, 1959–   . II. Title.
    RC423.R896   1999
    616.85'5—dc21   99-35810
                                                                CIP

Printed in the United States of America

10   9   8   7   6   5   4   3   2   1   03   02   01   00   99

CONTENTS

PREFACE

We have both been teaching speech science to undergraduate students for about five years now. While we love speech science and try to stimulate a similar interest in the young minds of future professionals, we were becoming increasingly dissatisfied with the available teaching materials. Every semester, we were also faced with well-founded complaints from students about the density of the reading and the difficulty grasping complicated concepts in acoustics without much background or preparation. An undergraduate speech science course may be a student's first exposure to speech acoustics.

It is probably true that many professors harbor a secret fantasy: that each and every one of their students go on for doctorates, become world-recognized experts in the field, and when beseiged by the media, gratefully acknowledge their professor's small, but significant, contribution in shaping that former student's brilliant career! But there has to be a starting place. We hope this text supplies that beginning step. In our judgment, most materials in the field tend to throw students "into the deep end" and not all students are naturally going to swim.

So, as the saying goes, when you want something done right, you do it yourself. It sounds simple *and* it makes sense. But we soon understood all too well the difficulty of breaking down complicated concepts into digestible portions. We quickly found ourselves walking a thin line between keeping the level of the material challenging enough to hold the interest of bright minds, and yet presenting facts clearly and simply enough in laying the foundations for the more complicated concepts.

We also felt it was extremely important to keep pointing out the relevance of speech science for students. Today's students are very goal-oriented. They lead busy lives and often have to balance part-time or even full-time jobs with their studies. Many future speech-language pathologists are also parents or attempting a change of career. They want to know how a course is relevant to their studies. We wanted to bring speech science "out of the laboratory and into the clinic." After all, the overwhelming majority of the students in our classes want to become speech-language pathologists and audiologists, not researchers. This is why we added to our title the qualifier "from basic theories to clinical applications"; we feel both theory and application are distinguishing features of our text.

We hope that we have achieved the right balance and that students will appreciate our efforts here. We have taken the approach that this book will not represent a student's only exposure to speech science, but rather in most cases his or her first exposure. As we know, however, first experiences are typically critical. If it is a pleasant experience, we have a much better chance of keeping the student for the longer distance—to graduate studies in the field.

We certainly have learned a lot from this experience and from interacting with students, and, just like our students, we hope to continue learning. We would like to thank the people at Allyn and Bacon, especially our editor Stephen D. Dragin, for their assistance and support of this project. We would also like to extend our gratitude to the outside reviewers for their time and thoughtful comments, which resulted in many improvements: Dennis Turner, Northern Arizona University; Jack Pickering, College of St. Rose; Lynn Chapman, University of Wyoming; and Dan Beasley, Memphis State University. Thanks also go to Kathy Whittier at Walsh & Associates, Inc. for her insightful copyediting of our manuscript. We dedicate this book to our students, past and future. We hope you'll enjoy this text.

CHAPTER

1 Introduction

Because as human beings we are verbal creatures, we surround ourselves with a verbal ocean. When we don't have live speech to listen to, we turn on the radio or television so we don't feel lonely. Or when there's no one else to talk to, we pick up the phone and call someone, making the distance between our conversational partner disappear. As verbal creatures, we are naturally curious about speech and language. Our ears strain to make out the message in a language we don't understand. Yet we feel compelled to try to comprehend anyway. People have been known to feign a foreign accent in an attempt to make themselves more interesting, while other people with natural accents try desperately to rid themselves of them. Speech is highly personal; it reveals who we are and who we would like to be.

Perhaps the most compelling evidence for the power of speech and language results from the devastating consequences to those fluent adults who suddenly lose the power of speech due to aphasia resulting from a stroke. Every one of us has felt tongue-tied at some point in our lives, and we have felt the frustration of not having our tongues obey what our brains are telling them to do. Imagine how difficult it would be to live in constant fear of stuttering. There is the slurred and difficult-to-understand speech of individuals with Parkinson disease and other neurogenic disorders. There is the concern of parents that their children might not be learning to speak at a normal pace, and the anguish of those who discover that their children are not speaking clearly because of a hearing loss. These are just some of the ways that speech can be affected; hopefully, part of the reason why you are in this course stems from a desire to help such people.

Speech science is the study of how speech is produced, how it is transformed into an acoustic signal, and what it is in this acoustic signal that listeners use to decode a verbal message. One major concern of speech science is measuring speech via both acoustic measures and physiological measures. Another concern of speech science is how the normal speech production process breaks down in various speech and language disorders.

This book is aimed primarily at the undergraduate student of speech-language pathology. It is intended to support the undergraduate course in speech science required by most programs in speech-language pathology and audiology.

1

To our knowledge, there are very few speech science texts written exclusively for an undergraduate readership. It is our experience that students' view of speech science is very much dependent on the introduction they receive to this area of inquiry. Students in speech science sometimes find themselves immersed in complicated acoustic concepts for which they have little or no preparation. They may even find speech science to be the most difficult material in their undergraduate program.

Unfortunately, bad experiences with speech science can be a deciding factor in deterring students from careers in speech-language pathology. This is indeed unfortunate, especially given the need for talented speech-language pathologists. It is our opinion that given sufficient introduction and preparation, students are capable of comprehending even the most intricate aspects of human speech. This book is meant to provide a nonthreatening, yet comprehensive, introduction to speech science.

Although designed first of all to serve an undergraduate student audience, this book is written in simple nontechnical language and would make an appropriate introduction for anyone who would like to learn more about the production of human speech. Speech is, after all, what makes us human, and learning more about speech is appropriate for the more general goal of understanding our species.

In addition, this text puts speech into its larger context of human language, speech after all being the spoken medium of language. It is our hope to prepare well-rounded speech-language pathologists and audiologists who will have been exposed to the rich linguistic abilities of humankind.

The present book need not be of interest only to the undergraduate speech-language pathology major. Concerned parents of children with speech disabilities should be able to gain a better understanding of their children's particular speech problem from this book. Hopefully, speech-language clinicians "out there in the field" will find this text a welcome refresher course on speech. Linguists and students of linguistic theory may likewise benefit from an introduction to the ins and outs of spoken language, vocal anatomy, and the acoustic and articulatory properties of a language's phonemic inventory. Finally, this book could serve as a condensed review of speech science for graduate students—either for the National Exam of Speech-Language Pathology and Audiology, or for the purposes of a graduate program's qualifying exams.

In the next chapter, we consider why it is necessary for students of speech-language pathology and audiology to have a thorough understanding of speech science. We know that students always want to know why they have to study something before they invest much time and effort into a particular subject matter. Hopefully, chapter 2 will provide a better understanding of why speech science courses are required at both the undergraduate and graduate level for certification by the American Speech-Language-Hearing Association.

The book is ordered along the traditional approach to speech in speech-language pathology with chapters on respiration (chapter 3), phonation (chapter 4), articulation (chapter 5), and resonance (chapter 6). These are the four basic processes of speech that are classic to speech-language pathology. Following these chapters is a brief discussion of phonology (chapter 7), the study of sound sequences in speech. Then, there are chapters on speech prosody (chapter 8), acoustic measures of speech (chapter 9), physiological measures of speech (chapter 10), and hearing (chapter 11). There is also a chapter on speech perception (chapter 12) so that students can better understand problems of speech that take their toll on the perceptual processes associated with speech. Speech production and speech perception are intimately related. The representation of speech in the brain is considered next (chapter 13). We then move to a discussion of how language evolved in chapter 14. Chapter 15 considers how a child develops a normal language system. Various speech and language disorders are discussed in chapter 16.

Because we find ourselves in the midst of the digital age, the computer is bound to play an increasing role in speech-language pathology and audiology. Computers and speech are discussed in chapter 17. Finally, chapter 18 considers speech science and the role of the speech-language pathologist in remediating speech. With this chapter, we hope to help future SLPs understand the professional role for which they are preparing themselves and to allow them to better comprehend their responsibilities as future health professionals.

We hope we have found an appropriate writing style for undergraduate students of speech science. We would like to "turn students on" to the rich and almost magical nature of speech, without "turning students off" with the jargon and complexity that could potentially overwhelm them. We tried to keep things simple, without condescension, to encourage developing professional knowledge. We have often referred to our own research work, certainly not because it is the only work available in a particular area, but rather because we would like to point out to students the relationship between teaching and research.

While every future speech-language pathologist owes it to him- or herself and to future clients to understand thoroughly the speech science that is basic to this profession, there is no rule against the slow and easy initiation that characterizes this text. Instead of alienating students, we hope to foster the love of speech and language that attracted them to this field in the first place.

Most students are capable of understanding even very complex and intricate processes, if they are given sufficient opportunity to understand the basics first. Hopefully, this book will provide just the right kind of basic groundwork for a very solid basis in the understanding of speech common to all effective speech-language pathologists.

You should look at your learning about speech science as a journey that will help you get to your destination of being a successful speech-language pathologist or audiologist. The trip may take a while, but there are a lot of interesting sights. We may even be able to have some fun together along the way. You'll be a somewhat different person when you arrive at your destination. We have tried to provide ample travel tips in the form of *Hints to Students* in places where our experience tells us that the going may be a little rough. And you'll find a glossary of key terms at the back of the text.

So welcome aboard. Sit back and relax, strap on your safety belts and let us wish you "Bon voyage!"

Why Speech-Language Pathologists Need to Study Speech Science

Sometimes it is not clear to students why a particular course is required for a particular degree. Understandably, students may lack motivation for a class whose relevance they question. It is important to understand why speech science is relevant and necessary for future speech-language pathologists (SLPs) and audiologists.

One of the primary motivations is that understanding a normal process is the first step towards understanding a disordered process. For example, one has to know that a car normally sits level in order to understand that something is wrong if the car is leaning to one side or the other.

One has to understand the normal speech process in order to know which component of the speech mechanism is disturbed in a particular disorder. Typically, speech therapy is directed as specifically as possible to the implicated speech processes. For example, it is important to know that articulation disorders usually involve the movement of the tongue and lips, while voice disorders involve the laryngeal mechanism. This distinction, as we shall see, relates directly to the source-filter theory of speech production whereby the vocal folds provide a sound source and the vocal tract acts as a filter to shape this sound into speech. But students must understand this distinction, otherwise they risk attempting voice therapy for articulation disorders and articulation therapy for voice disorders. Obviously, articulation therapy is not going to be very effective when the source of the problem is faulty laryngeal valving.

This chapter attempts to answer the question of why speech science is a required course for speech-language pathology majors. Some of the particular applications of speech measures are considered as they are applied in the field of speech-language pathology. The nine basic reasons for studying speech science are summarized in Table 2.1.

Understand Baseline Measures

Speech science allows the SLP to understand baseline measures of speech production and perception, against which pathologies can be compared. The normal

TABLE 2.1   Nine Basic Reasons for Future Speech-Language Pathologists to Study Speech Science

1. Understand baseline measures of speech
2. Keep abreast of technological advances in the field
3. Understand and meet the needs of bilingual clients
4. Facilitate second language acquisition
5. Reduce regional accents
6. Understand the link between speech production and speech perception
7. Promote greater sensitivity to language
8. Obtain and understand a universal perspective of the human species
9. Maintain and promote professionalism

functions (i.e., within a normal range of variation) of respiration, phonation, and vocal tract resonance comprise the very basic functions of human speech production. Understanding baseline values allows the SLP to differentiate between "different" and "abnormal" functioning, helping to ensure a more accurate diagnosis of speech disorders. Recent advances in our knowledge of how humans *perceive* speech sounds compared to nonspeech sounds also add to the SLP's basic education.

Speech science, then, provides SLPs with speech measures, in terms of the physiology of respiration, phonation, and articulation and the acoustic properties of speech (for example, the characteristics of a speech sound's frequency, amplitude, and duration). In turn, these measures can be used to assess the effectiveness of a particular therapy. As health management becomes more cost-conscious, it has become increasingly important to demonstrate the value of a particular intervention. SLPs are increasingly using speech measures to demonstrate the effectiveness of the therapy that they provide. Speech measures can provide an objective assessment of a client's improvement. These measures can provide feedback for clients who are trying to modify their speech production and evidence of progress. Indeed, the presence of speech science in the field of speech-language pathology bears directly on treatment.

Keep Abreast of Technological Advances in the Field

Recent advances in such technologies as digital spectrograms and Visipitch software for personal computers have allowed SLPs to use visual printouts of clients' speech as feedback in therapy. For example, clients are able to see a waveform of their own production and an "ideal" token of a certain speech sound as comparison. Some computer systems, such as IBM's SpeechViewer, allow clients to work on improving speech production in a video game-like format. Such technology also enables SLPs to work with clients on the melodic component of speech, such as changes in fundamental frequency over the length of a sentence and correct stressing of words and syllables, in addition to the accurate production of consonants and vowels.

To be able to interpret such visual data and use the equipment optimally, SLPs must have basic knowledge of acoustic and articulatory phonetics and be able to read spectrograms, spectra, and waveforms (which are all visual representations of speech). SLPs need to understand the theoretical concepts behind the speech exercises in order to use them properly.

Understand and Meet the Needs of Bilingual Clients

One of the largest growing populations of clients for SLPs is made up of bilingual speakers who seek dialect therapy. The advances in speech technology described above can again be employed when working with clients on articulation of consonants, vowels, and the melodic components of speech. Comparison of ideal tokens of speech sounds with clients' speech offers immediate feedback and provides the therapist important data.

Facilitate Second Language Learning

Often SLPs will be consulted by clients who are learning a second or foreign language as adults (different from bilingual speakers who learn two languages at the same time) and wish to improve their production of nonnative speech sounds or alter sentence intonation and speech melody to better approximate that of the target language. Here, SLPs can again assist with their knowledge of how speech sounds may differ between two languages and how production and perception of nonnative consonants and vowels change from childhood to adulthood. A basic knowledge of how speech is produced by the human vocal anatomy as well as the acoustic traits (i.e., physical properties) of speech sounds will allow an SLP to assist in a more informed way.

A touch more glamorous is the actor who seeks help from an SLP to master a foreign accent for a role. Meryl Streep is known for her intense practice of the speech sounds and accurate melody of her characters' native languages. SLPs can also assist professional speakers and singers to make more effective use of their voices and overcome various problems that they may encounter.

Reduce Regional Accents

Even monolingual clients who technically are not in need of speech therapy will sometimes seek therapy to reduce native accent traits or reduce regionalisms. We know of several respected colleges in New York City that offer adult education classes such as "How to Lose Your New York Accent." Without commenting on whether this "need" to lose one's regional speech traits is entirely justified, we include it here in this chapter as one of the ways SLPs can better serve their clients with a knowledge of language differences and speech science. Again, computer-generated speech tokens and auditory or visual feedback can help the therapist guide the client to his or her more desired pronunciation.

Be aware here that "accent" only refers to a particular *pronunciation* of speech sounds, that is, the phonetics and phonology of language. "Dialect" is the larger term and includes not only pronunciation, but also vocabulary choices, sentence structure, markers on nouns such as plural and possessive suffixes, verb tenses and variations in other levels of languages. Hence, even if a person loses an accent, he or she may still retain linguistic characteristics of a region or social class.

Understand the Link Between Speech Production and Speech Perception

The study of speech science allows the future SLP to see the close link between the production and perception of speech sounds—how the sounds the human vocal tract can produce are well-matched to the sounds that we can process with our auditory and neurological wiring. Speech is acoustically very complex, presented to the human listener rapidly and with overlapping clues to a particular sound's identification. Yet, we are able to understand speech with a high degree of accuracy. Furthermore, nonspeech sounds such as clicks, tones, and musical chords that are presented as rapidly as speech are not processed with nearly the same accuracy as speech perception. In addition, some evidence exists that other mammals can also process speech sounds such as consonants in a similar fashion to humans. This suggests that the auditory system of mammals in general may be a good processor for human speech.

The material covered in a speech science course treats speech production and speech perception as a part of an integrated system for which the anatomy of the human body has adapted over the course of evolution.

Promote Greater Sensitivity to Language

Speech-language pathology students need to be sensitive not only to speech but to language as well. Speech is often referred to as "spoken language," one of several channels by which human communication is transmitted. We believe it is essential that professionals in the field of speech understand and appreciate the larger concepts of human language, including the linguistic descriptions found in various linguistic theories and the processing mechanisms described in psycholinguistics.

In addition, we feel that it is important not to ignore the larger social framework in which speech and language exist. A speaker does not exist in a vacuum; he or she interacts in a social and cultural way with other speakers. This discussion reminds us of the question about the tree falling in the forest. If no one is there to hear the tree fall, does it still make a noise? Essentially for our purposes, if no one is there to perceive a person's speech, then no true speech act has occurred. Speech is produced in order to be perceived by a listener. We speak not simply to pacify ourselves with a comforting bath of linguistic babble, but rather for a specific purpose. We speak to be understood by, and to transmit specific information to, a listener.

The acoustic as well as the articulatory characteristics of speech would be better understood (and remembered) if students were aware of how these aspects relate to the phonetic features often used in the field. Simply memorizing facts cannot be as rewarding and long-lasting as actually understanding what those facts mean—the origin and logic behind them.

Obtain and Understand Universal Perspective of the Human Species

Speech science allows SLPs to see humans in a more universal context. As a species, we share many speech and language abilities, and we all have access to the same articulatory, anatomical, and neurological equipment. In other words, we share the biological bases of language. Although most of the time people tend to emphasize the wide differences among world languages, we feel that these differences may be outweighed by the similarities. While there are a lot of differences in the sounds used in various languages of the world, it is also remarkable that certain speech sounds are found over and over again in various languages. These sounds seem particularly well-suited for their role as units of speech.

Speech science provides a picture of speech in the world that is larger than just our species. What properties do we share with non-human primates and with mammals in general? As mentioned earlier, it seems that speech sounds may have evolved through the exploitation of the basic properties of the mammalian auditory system. The vocal tract of newborn humans is similar to that of mature non-human primates. Comparisons such as these work to place humans in a larger global context.

Maintain and Promote Professionalism

Finally, our goal is to contribute to the education of well-rounded speech-language pathology professionals. In this attempt, we treat our readers as future academics and researchers, as well as professionals. Speech science discusses what is currently known about human speech production and perception. It also alerts us to what still needs to be discovered and better understood in the processing of speech and language. As future professionals, you are invited to take part in the search for answers to these important questions. With your knowledge of speech science, training in a course of speech-language pathology, and through your contact with clients, you will possess the basic tools of research. Indeed, assessing the abilities of a client, providing therapy, and reporting on results are all part of clinical practice in speech-language pathology.

You owe it to your future clients to learn and understand as much as you can about the speech process that you will be called upon to remediate. Understanding speech science is an integral part of your responsibility as a speech-language pathologist or audiologist.

Study Questions

1. Without looking back at the text, name at least five reasons why SLPs need to study speech science.

2. You are an SLP in a hospital setting. There is a Health Maintenance Organization (HMO) threatening to no longer pay for speech-language services unless you can demonstrate the effectiveness of your therapy for your client. How does this chapter suggest that you might proceed to justify your therapy? (Hint: Of course you would have to have access to appropriate equipment.)

3. Do you think that you should help clients who want to get rid of their regional accents? Discuss the pros and cons of such therapy.

3 Respiration

Respiration is necessary to sustain life. It provides the oxygen required by all living tissues. The brain is one of the human organs whose supply of oxygen is most critical—the brain can only be deprived of oxygen for no more than a few precious minutes before permanent damage occurs.

In this chapter we will focus on respiration as it relates to speech production. Since there is an entire course devoted to anatomy and physiology in speech-language pathology programs, we will not consider them in detail in this chapter. Students interested in more detail on the anatomy and physiology of respiration are referred to Zemlin (1998).

The Nature of Breathing

Although the main role of respiration is to supply oxygen to the body, it is also required to produce speech. That is, respiration serves both a life-sustaining function and a speech-production function. We are all aware to some degree of the dependence of speech upon respiration. Popular sayings such as "talk until you're out of breath" or "say it until you're blue in the face" allude to this dependence of speech on breathing. We are also aware of the drive to finish one complete sentence on a single breath, even if it causes discomfort, and how odd it sounds when a speaker inadvertently inhales in the middle of a sentence. But there are several other more subtle ways in which the breathing used for speech is different than normal quiet breathing.

One of these differences is that while in quiet breathing a person spends just about equal time inhaling and exhaling; in breathing for speech, a person spends much more time exhaling than inhaling. Because we typically only produce speech on exhaled breath, speakers tend to spend only about 10 percent of a breath cycle inhaling and about 90 percent exhaling. This difference in the inspiration-to-expiration ratio between quiet breathing and breathing for speech is rather remarkable.

Hixon, Mead, and Goldman (1976) have shown that even though a person spends less time inhaling for speech than for quiet respiration, a greater volume of air is typically taken in. This suggests that speech is more effortful than quietly breathing, since a greater volume of air is exchanged for speech. The differences between quiet breathing and breathing for speech prove two points: first, that speech processes are built on more basic life-sustaining functions such as breathing, and second, that adaptations are made in such functions to accommodate speech. This difference may also be important because these two different functions of breathing may be controlled by somewhat different neurological structures.

Hint to Students

Inhale/exhale percentages for quiet breathing have been estimated at about 40%/60%, while for speech they are about 10%/90% (Borden, Harris, & Raphael, 1994). Initiating speech typically requires full lungs and sustained exhalation of air to continue speaking.

Respiration and Types of Sentences

There is evidence that speakers adjust their breathing to meet the requirements of the sentence they are about to produce. For example, speakers take in a greater volume of air when they have a longer sentence to produce. They may also adjust their intake to accommodate sentences that have more sounds requiring greater airflow, such as the /h/ sound, or more stress and emphasis on particular syllables.

Lieberman (1967) has hypothesized that a single sentence is usually spoken in a single *breath group*, which is characterized by a relatively steady fundamental frequency throughout the sentence with a fall-off in frequency at a sentence's terminal portion. The frequency pattern can be associated with a gradual decrease in air pressure below the vocal folds to allow exhalation and additional loss of subglottal pressure as one ends an utterance and forces the remaining air from the lungs. A fuller discussion on this can be found in chapter 8.

In one type of sentence, the rhetorical question, the rise or fall of the fundamental frequency distinguishes between a question and a statement. In these rhetorical questions, it is the rise of the fundamental frequency at the end of the sentence that signals that the speaker is asking a question instead of making a statement. Thus, if a speaker says "We're learning about respiration and speech" with a falling intonation, listeners know that a statement is being made. However, if the same words are produced with a rising intonation—"We're learning about respiration and speech?"—listeners know they are being asked a question. You can see this difference in Figures 3.1 and 3.2.

Lieberman (1967) has reviewed studies from a variety of different languages that all confirm that rising intonation contours result in questions, even in tone languages like Chinese in which pitch changes can signal different word meanings. To produce such rises in fundamental frequency at the end of a sentence, when air from the lungs is running out, is a somewhat tricky procedure. There are various ways to increase the pitch of your voice, and one of them is to increase the flow of

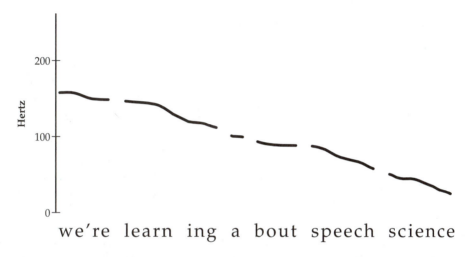

FIGURE 3.1   Schematic of a fundamental frequency contour for the statement "We're learning about speech science."

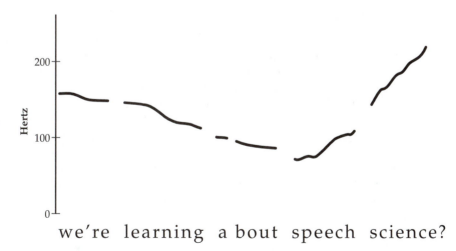

FIGURE 3.2   Schematic of a fundamental frequency contour for the question "We're learning about speech science?"

air from the lungs. If you use up too much air, toward the sentence's end you may not be able to achieve that pitch rise.

Speakers tend to produce the question versions of such question-statement pairs at significantly faster rates than the statement versions (Ryalls, Le Dorze, Lever, Ouellet, & Larfeuil, 1995). These researchers suggest that speakers produce the question version at a slightly faster rate in order to preserve the air that could help produce the rise in intonation at the end of the sentence. This is because the end of the sentence is where speakers typically have the lowest reserves of air left in their lungs.

Breathing for Speech

We will consider a few more ways in which breathing for speech is different, but readers should not get the impression that our treatment here is exhaustive. It is not yet entirely clear how breathing for speech is different from quiet breathing. More studies must be conducted that specifically investigate these differences. We encourage our readers to consider themselves researchers in the speech and language field. There are many questions left to answer in the discipline of speech science, and SLPs can sometimes gain new insights from data obtained from their clients.

Some of the most important differences in the breathing that occurs for speech, compared to quiet breathing, take place in the muscle activity. First, we will consider the muscle activity of inspiration and expiration in quiet breathing. To inhale, the body makes use of a property of physics whereby areas with different amounts of air pressure tend toward a balance. Air particles in an area of high air pressure will always try to move to an area of lower air pressure to even things out.

Inspiration

When we inhale, the air pressure within the lungs (also called *subglottal air pressure*) is relatively low compared to outside the lungs (*atmospheric air pressure*) and this condition allows air to rush in from the atmosphere. Certain physiological conditions must be met. First, the vocal folds must be open. Second, the air pressure in the lungs can be made even lower than outside to assist inspiration. This is done by increasing the space (volume) within the lungs. Another law of physics, Boyle's Law, states that volume and pressure are inversely related. Thus, if the volume of a given area is enlarged, the air pressure will fall. We want the lungs to increase their volume so the lower air pressure will encourage a good air flow into the lungs. The volume increase is achieved by lowering the diaphragm, which sits below the lungs and to which the lungs attach. They will lower and thus lengthen with the diaphragm. Meanwhile, the rib cage rises to increase lung volume in that dimension. The muscles between each rib (the intercostal muscles) work to raise the rib cage. In other words, the lungs are passive in inspiration.

Air will rush into the space with lower air pressure and continue to do so until air pressure above and below the vocal folds is equalized. This is the completion of inspiration and is roughly the same whether the individual is breathing to sustain life or preparing to talk. Remember, the main difference is that in speaking, a person will need to take in a greater volume of air. This can be done by increasing the volume of air in the lungs even more, causing a greater difference in air pressure on both sides of the vocal folds, and allowing a greater volume of air to enter the lungs.

Expiration

Expiration for quiet breathing and for speech, however, differs in muscle activity. For quiet exhalation, the ribs and diaphragm muscles are relatively inactive. Going back to physics, if the air pressure within the lungs is greater than above the vocal folds, air will move out of the lungs. The pressure differential can be achieved by decreasing the volume in the lungs, thereby increasing air pressure. The muscles originally used to increase volume are now relaxed, a passive maneuver whereby the diaphragm rises and the rib cage lowers, all decreasing the lung volume. Elastic recoil and other properties of muscular tissue allow the muscles to relax and return to a resting place. Thus, the air pressure has now been increased, and when it is higher than pressure above the vocal folds, air will rush out of the lungs.

Hint to Students

In respiration, volume changes, then pressure changes. An increase in volume gives you a decrease in pressure. Air moves from areas of high to low pressure to even things out.

Remember that a speaker devotes most of the respiratory cycle to exhaling and must use the amount of air wisely to last the entire duration of his or her utterance. In addition, if a question is produced requiring a pitch rise to the terminal portion of the intonation contour, the speaker might run out of air. Increasing subglottal air pressure not only increases fundamental frequency, but it also increases volume (heard as increased loudness). Because of lower lung volumes and the requirement to maintain fairly constant volume, the increase in fundamental frequency at the end of sentence is likely due to an increase in the tension in the vocal folds. It seems logical that the overall fall-off of fundamental frequency over the length of the sentence is likely due to decreasing subglottal air pressure resulting from lower lung volumes. But local increases in fundamental frequency, such as increases in fundamental frequency on certain words or parts of a sentence, are likely to be the result of increasing vocal fold tension.

Expiration for speech has three distinct stages. In the first stage, the muscles of inspiration continue to be active. This statement may seem contradictory, until we remember the reason for the continued activity of inspiratory muscles in the first stages of expiration. Inspiratory muscles apparently continue to be active in the first moments of expiration to provide a "braking" force. That is, the muscles of inspiration prevent the lungs from collapsing very quickly and the air from rushing out just as quickly as it was taken in. Remember that a speaker typically only uses 10 percent of the respiratory cycle for inspiration and has to stretch out this inhaled air for the other 90 percent of the time in speech.

In the second stage of expiration for speech, the muscles of inspiration cease activity, and the natural elastic recoil of the lungs now accounts for the air being exhaled. This is the stage of expiration for speech that is most similar to normal quiet exhalation. At this stage, the air coming from the lungs is very similar to air rushing out of a balloon.

In the third and final stage of expiration for speech, the muscles of expiration typically come into play. The muscles of expiration serve to squeeze out the remaining air to keep the pressure more equal over the whole length of the sentence. This stage is similar to squeezing on the sides of a balloon to keep air coming out at a more constant rate. Without squeezing the sides of the balloon, the rate at which air would come out of the balloon would slow down more and more as the balloon returned to its uninflated state.

Hint to Students

For the three stages of exhalation for speech, think (1) inspiratory muscles, (2) elastic recoil, (3) expiratory muscles.

Expiration for speech, then, has these three distinct stages with different muscle activity, in contrast to quiet breathing, which is mostly accounted for by the passive forces such as the natural elastic recoil of the lungs. One quickly understands that breathing for speech is more complicated and requires more coordinated muscle activity than quiet breathing. We should also consider that some sounds of speech require more air to produce than other sounds, and that speakers usually emphasize different words of a sentence by producing some words more loudly or softly than other words. We begin to appreciate just how complicated it probably is for speakers to structure their breathing to accommodate speech. Yet we are not typically even aware of greater effort required for speech. It is only when we attempt to speak during some very strenuous physical activity (e.g., while jogging or lifting a heavy package) that we even appreciate how constrained speech is by respiration.

Respiration and Disorders

We should also briefly consider how some disorders affect speech by changing respiration. For example, persons with Parkinson disease typically produce speech that is much softer than typical speech. This speech is often less distinguishable to listeners, and sometimes the words seem garbled or less clearly articulated.

But speakers with Parkinson disease often produce speech at a faster-than-normal rate—exactly the opposite of what would seem to be logical if their speech is less intelligible to listeners. However, this faster speech production gives us a clue that speakers with Parkinson disease may also be experiencing shortness of breath. In other words, the disease may compromise the efficient use of air for speech. Although not yet specifically investigated, it is tempting to speculate that these patients may unconsciously be speeding up their production in an attempt to compensate for their inefficient use of air.

Many times, SLPs have reported anecdotally that encouraging patients to have better posture and take deeper breaths has a natural beneficial effect on speech production. In fact, this connection is the basis of the Alexander Technique, a body-realignment program started by an actor who kept losing his voice during performances. Matthias Alexander discovered a correlation between voice amplitude and body posture.

In other words, improved breathing may result in more intelligible speech. Borden and colleagues (1994) suggest that oftentimes what appears to be a lack of breath turns out rather to be a case of poor use of the breath. Certainly, Ramig, Bonitati, Lemke, and Horii (1994) have shown that Parkinson patients can benefit thoroughly from a program of respiratory and vocal exercise that they have developed. Named after a particularly inspiring patient, the Lee Silverman Method has given many patients a new lease on life through improved speech intelligibility.

It is important that students of speech-language pathology be aware of the intimate relationship that respiration has with speech production. We can have the most inspirational message in the world, with just the right choice of words. But it won't do us much good if we don't have the breath to say it.

Study Questions

1. Explain the process that allows air to enter the lungs.

2. Explain how breathing to sustain life is different from breathing for speech.

3. What does research about the production of sentence intonation contours add to our knowledge of breathing for speech?

4. How do data from neurologically impaired individuals add to such knowledge?

References

Borden, G., Harris, K., & Raphael, L. (1994). *Speech primer* (3rd ed.). Baltimore: Williams and Wilkins.

Hixon, T., Mead, J., & Goldman, M. (1976). Dynamics of the chest wall during speech production: Function of the thorax, rib cage, diaphragm, and abdomen. *Journal of Speech and Hearing Research, 19*, 297–356.

Lieberman, P. (1967). *Intonation, perception and language.* Cambridge, MA: MIT Press.

Ramig, L., Bonitati, C., Lemke, J., & Horii, Y. (1994). Voice treatment for patients with Parkinson's disease: Development of an approach and preliminary efficacy data. *Journal of Medical Speech-Language Pathology, 2,* 191–209.

Ryalls, J., Le Dorze, G., Lever, N., Ouellet, L., & Larfeuil, C. (1995). The effect of age and sex on speech intonation and duration. *Journal of the Acoustical Society of America, 95,* 2274–2276.

Zemlin, W. (1998). *Speech and hearing science* (4th ed.). Boston: Allyn & Bacon.

4 Phonation

We saw in chapter 3 on respiration that many anatomical structures and functions necessary to speech production have more basic life-sustaining functions. This is also true for the vocal folds. Phonation refers to the vibration of the vocal folds.

The Vocal Folds

Although the primary function of the vocal folds is to act as a valve for the lungs and protect them from the aspiration of food and other substances into the lungs, they are also essential for the production of speech. Sometimes they are referred to as the "vocal cords." However, they are attached along one side and do not vibrate freely like a cord, so we will use the preferred term *vocal folds*.

The vocal folds can be approximated tightly to keep air inside of the lungs and make the thorax (chest cavity) rigid and provide a basis of support for lifting heavy objects. (You might have guessed that the vocal folds were somehow involved in lifting heavy weights from the grunts of weightlifters or the sound that some tennis players make when their racquets make contact with the ball.)

Everyone is familiar with the role that the vocal folds play in expelling substances out of the lungs by coughing. Coughing is a rapid release of subglottal air pressure that can be made intentionally or unintentionally. The purpose of a cough is to blow substances such as mucus away from the entrance to the lungs. We take such a basic act as coughing for granted. However, persons with *dysphagia* (a disorder of swallowing) may not be able to cough properly, making them much more susceptible to choking and pneumonia due to aspiration of food or liquid into the lungs. Indeed, our entire species is vulnerable to choking because the openings to the lungs and to the stomach are relatively close together. "Talking with your mouth full" may result in an opened trachea *and* esophagus, and many people have died from food passing down the wrong tube.

In contrast, no other species has such an accident-prone vocal anatomy, and even human infants start with a safer vocal design than adult humans. The payoff for having our vocal folds close to the opening to the esophagus, though, is that our entire vocal tract is larger due to a lower larynx. Because of the nearly right-angle bend in the modern human's vocal tract, we can better isolate two independently resonating cavities (one oral and the other pharyngeal) and thus produce more and better speech sounds. Some of the speech sounds that are allowed by the human vocal tract are particularly acoustically stable sounds. These sounds are referred to as *quantal*. Quantal sounds allow for faster speech production because they can be articulated with relative imprecision with little change in their acoustic structure.

When the vocal folds are placed under just the right conditions—they are approximated firmly but not too tightly—they can vibrate rapidly. It is this rapid vibration of the vocal folds that we hear as "voice." You can feel this vibration by humming and placing your fingers on your larynx (or "voice box"). Because males have somewhat larger larynges, this area of the throat is a little more prominent on males, where it is called the "Adam's apple."

There are actually two senses of the term *voice*. One is nontechnical and refers to the individual sound quality of a particular person when he or she speaks. The other more technical sense of the term refers to the sound that the vocal folds make when they vibrate. This latter sense of the term refers to the vibrating sound source for many speech sounds.

Fundamental Frequency

The rate at which the vocal folds vibrate is referred to as the *fundamental frequency*. Fundamental frequency is often abbreviated as f_0 (pronounced f-oh, or f-zero). Fundamental frequency is usually perceived as a person's vocal pitch, so a lower f_0 value is heard as a deeper voice. Most women and all children have higher f_0 values, which listeners hear as higher-pitched voices. It should be pointed out, however, that the vocal folds are constantly changing in fundamental frequency from when they first begin to vibrate, as the speaker places more emphasis on certain words and as the vocal folds slow down for the end of a sentence.

Hint to Students

Fundamental frequency refers to the actual rate of vibration of the vocal folds, while pitch refers to the perception of fundamental frequency by human listeners.

Hint to Students

Originally the symbol for the fundamental frequency was f_0 (the integral sign, sub-zero). However, probably because of typesetting limitations, the capital F symbol with a zero (F_0), or Fø, has become the standard in most texts. This is somewhat unfortunate, because it makes it much easier for students to confuse the fundamental frequency with formant frequencies which are written F_1, F_2, F_3, etc. Since, as we will see, there is no relationship between the fundamental frequency and formant frequencies, even though both are frequency measures expressed in Hertz, we will return to the use of f_0 in this text. We will do this even though students should be aware that many other texts use F_0.

So even though a single average value is typically used to describe the fundamental frequency, you should be aware that the rate of vibration of the vocal folds is not static but rather is constantly changing. Typically this rate of vibration is measured in Hertz. *Hertz*, abbreviated Hz, has replaced the older term cycles per second or c.p.s. There is one Hertz for each cycle or each complete opening and closing of the vocal folds per second. So for an adult male voice with a fundamental frequency of 100 Hz, the vocal folds open and close completely 100 times in one second (although this value is a little low for a typical male voice; perhaps 120 Hertz is a more typical value). An average adult female might have a fundamental frequency of 200 Hz, so her vocal folds would open and close completely 200 times per second.

Hint to Students

Like the speed of driving a car in miles per hour, the vocal folds vibrate at different rates in Hertz. Even though the average speed of an automobile may be 40 miles per hour, we constantly have to slow down and speed up again at traffic lights. Similarly, there are voiceless sounds in most sentences that require the vocal folds to momentarily stop vibrating.

For a child, the vocal folds may vibrate at 300 times per second (i.e., 300 Hz) or higher. Although there is no single agreed upon average values for each gender, these are mnemonically convenient values—100 Hz for men, one octave (an octave is a doubling of frequency) higher at 200 Hz for women, and another 100 Hz higher for infants at 300 Hz.

Hint to Students

Larger structures vibrate more slowly than smaller structures. Think of larger, thicker vocal folds taking longer to complete one cycle of phonation.

It should be pointed out here that even though there are some differences in the typical fundamental frequency (rate of vibration of the vocal folds) for inherent differences in the vocal folds and laryngeal structure due to age and gender, it is not these differences that account for the differences between the various sounds of speech. The fundamental frequency can remain the same for a whole series of vowel sounds produced by the same speaker. The simple sound of the vibrating vocal folds is modified through resonance and molded into the various sounds of speech. This process of resonance is considered in the next chapter.

In order for the vocal folds to vibrate, the speaker must have *inspired* or taken sufficient air into the lungs. Remember that one takes in more air during an inspiration that is going to be used for speech than would be the case in quiet breathing.

When breathing quietly, a person typically spends about equal time inspiring (breathing in) and expiring (breathing out). But a person who is speaking typically spends as little as 10 percent of the breathing cycle in inspiration and as much as 90 percent or more breathing out. This is understandable since, in almost all cases, speech is produced during expiration—what is called an *egressive flow of air*. Although it is possible to produce some speech on inspiration (the inward or *ingressive flow of air*), this is usually very rare. In some languages, speakers may communicate the last unit of a series of items on inward flow of air in order to emphatically signal the end. Or they may do so in order to emphasize certain words.

It is interesting to observe just how skilled speakers are at coordinating respiration and speech, since they rarely (almost never) run out of breath before the end of a sentence. Lieberman and Lieberman (1973) found that people have an idea of the length of their intended utterance and inspire accordingly. Speakers typically only take breaths in between sentences, and they may even produce two or three sentences on the same breath. There are various forms of evidence that have been used to demonstrate the rather intricate control of breathing when its purpose is speech. (Recall from the previous chapter that speakers tend to produce questions that require a rise in fundamental frequency at a faster rate than statements that do not require the rise.)

The Anatomy of Phonation

Before detailing the process of phonation, we must briefly review the anatomy of the larynx, which is the series of cartilages, muscles, and tendons that make up and surround the vocal folds. The vocal folds are associated with three main cartilaginous structures and muscles that either close the vocal folds, open them, or tighten them. A speaker may increase tension on the vocal folds in order to raise the rate of vocal fold vibration, and hence raise the f_o.

As can be seen in Figure 4.1, the three main cartilages of the larynx are the *thyroid cartilage*, the *cricoid cartilage*, and a pair called the *arytenoid cartilages*.

We will discuss each in turn. The thyroid cartilage looks like a shield with the fuller section in front and tapered section in back. At the front, this shield arches, and for men this arch is at a more acute angle than for women. The male Adam's apple, prominent on men's throats, results from the notch of the thyroid cartilage. Women have Adam's apples in a way, in that there is still a thyroid notch, but it is not as acute in women, and hence less pronounced.

Hint to Students

The thyroid cartilage is like a shield; the cricoid like a ring; and the arytenoids are like triangles.

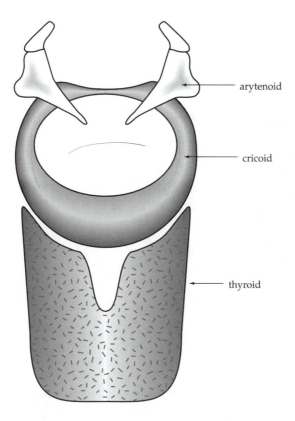

FIGURE 4.1   Schematic diagram of the three main cartilages of the larynx.

Above the thyroid is the cricoid cartilage, which is shaped like a signet, or school ring. Unlike a ring, though, the fuller section is found in back and the thinner part anterior to (in front of) the larynx.

Sitting on top of the cricoid are the two triangular shaped arytenoid cartilages. They can rotate inward and outward when certain muscles are tensed. Generally, all parts of the larynx and the structure move as a whole, mainly up and down. The structure known as the vocal folds stretches from the arytenoids to the inside of the thyroid cartilage. Because of this, the movement of the whole larynx may result in a higher fundamental frequency. Specifically, the vocal folds attach to an angle of the arytenoid called the *vocal process*. The folds themselves are composed of muscles, tendons, and ligaments.

There are five main muscles that alter the placement of the vocal folds. The names of these muscles will help you remember where they are located, and vice versa. The three cartilages and these muscles all work together to prepare the vocal folds to vibrate, remain still, or tense for the purposes of increasing voice pitch. These muscles are illustrated in Figure 4.2. Although there is not complete

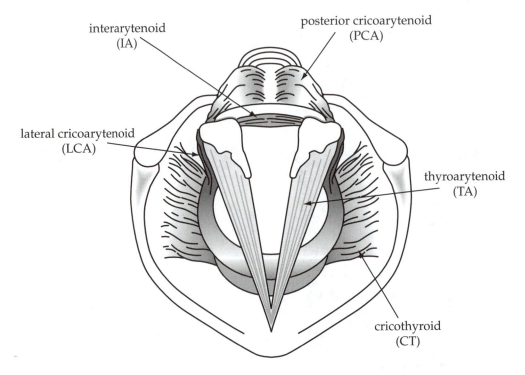

FIGURE 4.2   Schematic diagram of the major muscles of the larnyx for adjusting fundamental frequency.

agreement in the scientific literature on exactly what muscles are responsible for which laryngeal adjustments, the summary that follows is consistent with most accounts.

The Process of Phonation

Closing the vocal folds is called *adduction*. The *interarytenoid muscle* runs between the two parts of the arytenoid cartilage. When muscles are tensed, they shorten. Tensing the interarytenoid muscle will pull the two triangles of the arytenoid cartilage together. This maneuver also brings the vocal folds closer together.

A secondary adducting muscle is the *lateral cricoarytenoid muscle*. Some speech sounds—for example, stop consonants—require a great deal of intraoral pressure. That is, they need air pressure in the oral cavity (mouth) to be great, with no leakage. An extra tight vocal fold adduction helps seal off the pharyngeal cavity. In such a case, both adduction muscles would be employed. The lateral cricoarytenoid muscle is located on the sides (lateral) of the cricoid and stretches to the arytenoids. When this muscle tenses, the shortened lateral cricoarytenoid pulls a corner of the arytenoid triangle (the muscular processes) forward, thus rotating both cartilages of the arytenoid. This rotation movement pulls the vocal processes closer; since the vocal folds are attached, they too approximate.

Pulling the vocal folds apart is called *abduction*. The *posterior cricoarytenoid muscle* is attached in the back (posterior) between the cricoid cartilage and the muscular processes of the arytenoid cartilages. When tensed, this muscle rotates the muscular processes inward and closer together. The vocal processes thus separate; consequently, the vocal folds also separate.

Tensing the vocal folds involves a primary and a secondary muscle. When a mass is pulled taut, it is thinner at any specific point and will thus vibrate more quickly. This is one way to increase the fundamental frequency (heard as pitch) of one's voice. To raise the fundamental frequency, the *cricothyroid muscle* can be employed. This structure connects between the cricoid and thyroid cartilages and when used will actually rock the cricoid back, pulling the arytenoids with it. The vocal folds tense up as a consequence, affecting the fundamental frequency, which increases.

The *thyroarytenoid muscle* is a secondary tensing muscle. This muscle, also called the *vocalis*, runs the length of the vocal folds themselves, between the thyroid and arytenoid cartilages. When tensed, this muscle works to decrease the vibrating mass of the vocal folds. Consequently, vibration actually increases. Remember, a thinner object can move more quickly, and the tensed vocal folds are technically thinner, although they also increase slightly in length.

Hint to Students

Primary and secondary muscles altering vocal fold placement and tension can be remembered as follows: abduction by posterior cricoarytenoid (PCA); adduction by interarytenoid (IA), with additional closure by lateral cricoarytenoid (LCA); tensing by cricothyroid (CT), with additional tensing by thyroarytenoid (TA).

The fundamental frequency can actually be affected in four ways by various processes. We have already discussed two ways to increase tension along the vocal folds in order to increase f_o. Primarily we can employ the cricothyroid muscle, and secondarily the thyroarytenoid muscle. We can also increase fundamental frequency by increasing subglottal air pressure. When a greater discrepancy exists between air pressure below the vocal folds and above the vocal folds, they will be blown farther apart. This will increase intensity or loudness. So amplitude and f_o rise together when subglottal air pressure is increased.

However, these two acoustic parameters can be manipulated separately. As a matter of fact, studies have shown that people stress syllables with individually varying combinations of amplitude, f_o, and duration manipulation, sometimes using all three or only one correlate to signal stress in a word (Behrens, 1988; Lieberman, 1960).

Hint to Students

Speakers can alter amplitude and fundamental frequency independently, so that an increase in one can, but need not, be accompanied by an increase in the other.

Finally, speakers can lower their f_o by lowering the entire laryngeal structure. This movement adds mass to the vocal folds and can be executed with the help of strap muscles in the neck.

The vocal folds are apart to let in the free flow of oxygen during inspiration. They must be drawn together or approximated (also called *adduction*) in order for them to begin vibrating.

Hint to Students

To remember adduction versus abduction, think of **add**ing as a process of putting things together, in this case, the vocal folds; while a person who is **abd**ucted is carried away.

Because the vocal folds are closed, air pressure builds up under the vocal folds. When this subglottal air pressure reaches a certain critical level, so that it is greater than above the glottis (i.e., supraglottal), the vocal folds are pushed apart and the air pressure from beneath then escapes.

Two forces act together to bring the vocal folds back together again for the cycle of vocal fold vibration to begin once more. First of all, the vocal folds are made up of resilient muscle and ligament material—that is, they are inherently elastic. Something elastic that is stretched has a tendency to return to its natural unstretched position. But there is also an aerodynamic principle, called the *Bernoulli force*, that acts to draw the vocal folds back together again. Simply put, the Bernoulli force is created from the release of air pressure when the vocal folds are first blown apart. The air rushes out faster, and this drop in pressure between the vocal folds causes the suction-like Bernoulli force, resulting in vocal fold adduction. In an airplane it is actually the Bernoulli force that causes the plane to lift off the ground. The Bernoulli force results from air pressure being greater under the wing of an airplane than over the wing since the air underneath is rushing by faster. The design of the wing makes it such that the air has a longer distance to travel under the wing than over the wing. This, in turn, causes wings to lift a plane off the ground.

You may also experience the effects of the Bernoulli force when driving close to the rear of a fast-moving truck and feeling your car being pulled toward it. But for speech purposes, you simply need to understand that the drop in air pressure caused by the opening of the vocal folds also creates the Bernoulli suction force that helps to bring them back together again.

These two forces that serve to bring the vocal folds back together again—one muscular-elastic, the other aerodynamic in nature—explain why this account of vocal fold activity is termed the *myoelastic aerodynamic* theory of vocal fold vibration.

Hint to Students

myo= muscle, elastic= elastic recoil, aero= air, dynamic= movement.

A somewhat more detailed account of vocal fold vibration takes into account that the vocal folds are not one undifferentiated mass; rather, there are layers to the vocal folds. The vibration of the vocal folds is more accurately represented by a model in which there is a stiffer body that is covered by a more flexible cover. Hence this model is known as the *cover-body theory of vocal fold vibration* (Hirano & Kakita, 1985)

There are also many fine details of vocal fold vibration, such as whether the vocal folds are entirely closed along their edge or whether a small gap or "chink" remains, giving a person's voice its individual character. It is rather amazing to think that there are enough individual differences in vocal fold vibration (along with other speech processes) to give voices their individual identity. We are usually able to recognize a voice over the telephone, even one that we haven't heard in years. And, of course, we can recognize the voices of all sorts of people we interact with on an infrequent basis. We often take this ability in listeners for granted and do not always bother to state our name to a close friend or relative over the phone: "Hi, it's me."

It only makes sense that individual voice recognition had a survival value in early humans, which may explain just how developed voice recognition is in our species. There is also evidence that this skill emerges very early in life, and many would argue that at least a part of voice recognition is innate. It's otherwise difficult to explain why a newborn infant shows a preference for its parents' voices from the time of birth. Certainly some of the individual acoustic character of a voice can be carried through the amniotic fluid of the womb to the ears of the developing fetus, but the fact that the future child knows what to listen for suggests innate genetic support for this process. More about the emergence of language abilities in infants can be found in chapter 15.

SLPs have to understand phonation in order to serve their clients with various voice disorders. Problems in voice can range from the simple temporary hoarse voice resulting from a cold or vocal abuse (such as extensive shouting at a sporting event or cheerleaders who tend to shout while performing strenuous physical exertion, perhaps one of the quickest routes to vocal problems) to more complex problems such as vocal nodules (which prevent the vocal folds from closing completely), to laryngeal cancer and even removal of the laryngeal mechanism (known as a laryngectomy). SLPs also treat secondary problems of laryngeal valving such as can occur in swallowing disorders. Some of the methods for observing the activity of the vocal folds is considered in chapter 10 on physiological measures of speech.

In the next two chapters, we will discuss how air from the lungs, after encountering the vocal folds, passes through the array of human articulators and cavities of the vocal tract to resonate and result in speech.

Study Questions

1. How are the vocal folds adjusted to produce voiced sounds? To produce voiceless sounds?

2. How may speakers increase their fundamental frequency? How may they increase voice amplitude? Explain the ways these two acoustic correlates are related.

References

Behrens, S. (1988). The role of the right hemisphere in the production of linguistic stress. *Brain and Language, 33*, 104–127.

Hirano, M., & Kakita, Y. (1985). Cover-body theory of vocal fold vibration. In R. G. Daniloff (Ed.), *Speech science*. San Diego, CA: College Hill Press.

Lieberman, P. (1960). Some acoustic correlates of word stress in American English. *Journal of the Acoustical Society of America, 32*, 451–454.

Lieberman, M., & Lieberman, P. 1973. Olson's "projective verse" and the use of breath control as a structural element. *Language and Style, 5*, 287–298.

5 Articulation and Phonetics

Articulation refers to the involvement of particular anatomical structures, collectively called articulators, to create the sounds of speech. Some articulators—such as the tongue, lips, and jaw—move to produce speech, while other articulators are the site of contact or near-contact for a second articulator, that is, where an articulator moves to. These sites or *places of articulation* include the teeth and sections of the area most people call the roof of the mouth.

Besides place of articulation, speech sounds are also classified by the manner in which they are produced: Is the air that flows from the lungs obstructed during production? Does the air flow through the oral or nasal cavity? These classifications are termed *manners of articulation*. Finally, a speech sound can be produced with the vocal folds vibrating or still, another feature of speech called *voicing*.

In this chapter, we look at phonetics, the study of speech sounds, in order to describe sounds by the phonetic features designating place and manner of articulation and voicing (for vowels, the features are a bit different, as we will see later). A phonetic symbol is traditionally used to denote each combination of features, a symbol that relates to one, and only one, speech sound. Such symbols form the International Phonetic Alphabet (IPA), and we will introduce the reader to the symbols associated with English consonants and vowels.

The IPA for both consonant and vowel sounds strives for an invariant relationship between the sound and the symbol. In English the sound "ee" as in *see* can be spelled quite a number of ways: "ea" as in *sea*, "eo" as in *people*, "i" as in *ski*. In contrast, the IPA designates a single symbol for the same sound, regardless of spelling. At times the IPA symbol and the spelled, or orthographic symbol, coincide. Sometimes they do not, so an "s" sound in English and an "s" sound in

Hint to Students

The IPA is based on sound, not spelling. Pay attention to the sounds of words rather than their spelling.

German are denoted by the same symbol. If an "s" in German is pronounced like a "z" sound, for example, it will be represented with an appropriate corresponding IPA symbol. Spelling interference is one trap that students learning phonetics often fall into, like writing [cæt] for *cat*.

Hint to Students

Brackets denote phonetic symbols, as opposed to alphabetic characters, associated with a particular speech sound. For example, even though the word *cat* is written with the letters "c," "a," and "t," it is written [kæt] in phonetic transcription. A [k] is used because the letter "c" here represents the sound [k]. In other words such as *cellar*, the "c" represents the sound [s].

Phonetics can be approached from an articulatory point of view, in which the physiological maneuvers of the articulators are the main focus of interest. Students can also learn about phonetics via the acoustic properties of speech. Known as acoustic phonetics, this approach examines the properties of duration, frequency, and amplitude of sounds, usually making use of visual depictions of speech such as waveforms, spectrograms, and spectra (see chapter 9 for a fuller discussion). Finally, phonetics may be studied as a perceptual phenomenon, by which the processing of speech sounds by listeners is examined, often with the goal of understanding what makes each speech sound unique to the human perceptual system and where and why confusion between sounds exists.

In this chapter, we mainly examine speech from an articulatory vantage point in order to associate each sound with an articulatory maneuver. In fact, the IPA is largely based on articulatory properties (Ladefoged, 1993). Later we will briefly look at several acoustic properties of consonants and vowels, shifting to an acoustic-phonetic analysis of speech.

Consonants

Place of Articulation

For consonants, articulators make contact or near-contact at a certain place in the vocal tract, and the airstream is modulated in various ways. Think of the vocal tract (VT) as all the passages and structures above the vocal folds. This term will help you to differentiate between harmonics and formant frequencies in the next section. The VT is also called the "supralaryngeal vocal tract" or sometimes the "supraglottal vocal tract."

Hint to Students

The space between the vocal folds is called the glottis; supraglottal or supralaryngeal refers to the vocal tract (VT), which is above the vocal folds.

The VT has three cavities (spaces): the oral cavity (mouth), the nasal cavity (nasal passages and sinuses), and the pharyngeal cavity (back of throat). These spaces are not actually empty—they are filled with the air particles that propagate sound. The displacement of air allows the sounds of speech to travel.

Included in the VT are the articulators. Of all possible combinations of maneuvers among these articulators, human languages use only a subset of sounds in their phonetic inventories. It seems to be the case that only sounds that are relatively easy to produce, and that are also easily distinguished by listeners, are used in the world's languages.

Some articulators you will already be familiar with: the lips, the tongue, the teeth. Other articulators, or places of articulation in this case, you may already know by their more informal terms: "roof of the mouth," "back of the throat," and so on. We will divide the roof of the mouth or *palate* into three areas: (1) the rigid area behind the teeth, called the *alveolar ridge*; (2) the arched and bony area forming the main part of the roof of the mouth, or the *hard palate*; and (3) the softer area behind the arch, or the *soft palate* (also called the *velum*). The velum is extended back into a flap-like structure (seen in the mouths of screaming cartoon characters as a punching bag) called the *uvula*. Finally, sounds produced at the glottis are considered glottal sounds.

These, then, are the places of articulation, where the consonant sounds of speech are produced. Each place has an associated adjective, so sounds produced at the velum are *velar*; at the alveolar ridge, *alveolar*; and at the hard palate, *palatal*.

More than one type of sound can be produced at the same place of articulation. Both [d] and [n] are alveolar sounds, but in the former, the airstream is actually stopped for a moment, then released in a burst; whereas the latter sound is formed by stopping the air in the oral cavity while giving it free passage through the nasal cavity. [s] is also an alveolar sound, but it is produced a third way. In fricative sounds like [s], the airstream is forced through a narrow constriction formed by the tongue approaching the alveolar ridge without making contact.

These different ways of creating speech sounds are termed manners of articulation. We thus need to specify not only place of articulation but manner of articulation as well when defining consonants.

Manner is traditionally listed starting with the sounds created with the most constriction in the oral cavity—occlusives such as stops and nasals—and ending with those produced with relatively little obstruction of the airstream—resonants such as liquids and glides. See Figure 5.1 for a summary of phonetic features for English consonants. The terms in the figure are defined below. We now turn to a discussion of manner of articulation.

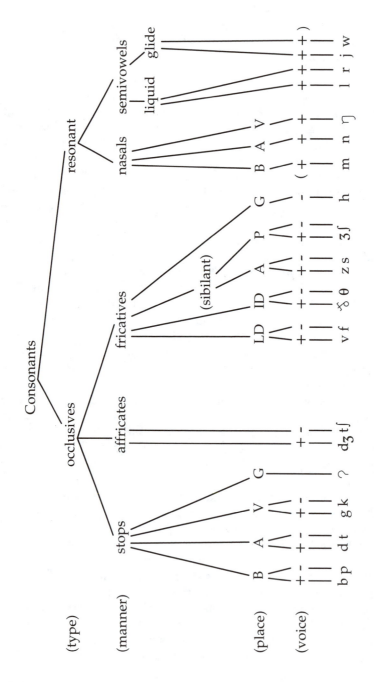

FIGURE 5.1 Chart of the consonants of American English arranged by type, manner, place, and voicing. B = bilabial, A = alveolar, V = velar, G = glottal, LD = lingua dental, ID = interdental, A = alveolar, P = palatal. (Reprinted with permission by Singular Publishing Group, Inc. from J. Ryalls, *A Basic Introduction to Speech Perception*, 1996.)

Manner of Articulation

Stops. In stop consonants, the airstream is stopped completely in the VT, then released all at once producing a puff of air or "burst." For English, there are stops produced with the constriction of the lips (bilabial: [p] & [b]); with the tip of the tongue reaching the alveolar ridge (alveolar: [t] & [d]); and with the dorsum (back) of the tongue at the velum (velar: [k] & [g]). (It is somewhat traditional to present speech sounds in the voiceless/voiced pairs in this manner.) In addition, there is a stop produced at the glottis, the glottal stop, [ʔ], as may be heard in Cockney English pronunciations as the "hiccup-like" sound in the middle of words such as *bottle* and *button*.

Some stops are produced without the release of air, usually when they occur at the end of a word. These differences in pronunciation will be discussed in chapter 7.

Nasals. The air is stopped completely in the oral cavity, but the nasal cavity is open for air to flow unobstructed. Some texts actually call these sounds "nasal stops" (Ladefoged, 1993), but we prefer to reserve the word "stop" for sounds produced with complete air stoppage. With the blockage at the lips, one produces the bilabial nasal [m]. When the tongue makes contact with the alveolar ridge, while air flows through the nasal cavity, the nasal [n] is produced. Finally, oral blockage at the velum produces the velar nasal [ŋ], as in the "ng" of *ring*. Notice that the placement of the tongue for the nasals is identical to the placement for the stops mentioned above (i.e., bilabial, alveolar, and velar), the only difference being in the manner of articulation: opened or closed nasal cavity.

Fricatives. In fricatives, the airstream is forced through a narrow passage formed by two articulators approximating each other, but not making contact. The turbulent sound that results is called *frication*. English fricatives are produced in several ways: (1) with the lower lip approximating the upper teeth, [f], [v]; (2) the tongue and alveolar ridge creating a narrow passage for the airflow, [s], [z]; (3) the tongue near the palate for the initial sound in the word *shoe* [ʃ] and the medial sound in *measure* [ʒ]; (4) and constriction at the glottis produces [h]. In addition, fricatives produced with more amplitude and high-frequency energy are categorized as sibilants [s, z, ʃ, ʒ]. The nonsibilant fricatives [f, v, θ, ð] are lower in amplitude and have no distinguishing high-frequency component.

Hint to Students

For fricatives, think *friction noise*.

Affricates.   For affricates, the air is stopped completely in the VT, then released into a narrow passage, to create a fricative. Affricates, then, share characteristics with both stops and fricatives, and they are sometimes denoted by a two-symbol phonetic character representing this combination (i.e., [tʃ] & [dʒ]). English affricates are both at the alveo-palatal region. (Note that texts vary on the designation of this place of articulation, some describing it as the "alveo-palatal" region, others simply as "palatal.") The affricates are [tʃ] as in *cheer* and [dʒ] as in *jeer*. Notice that the stop half of both sounds is alveolar, while the fricative part is palatal, perhaps leading to the disagreement in terminology for place.

The following two types of speech sounds, liquids and glides (as well as nasals), are always voiced, so they do not come in voiced/voiceless pairs like the previous speech sounds. They are sometimes referred to collectively as semivowels, since they assume relatively little VT constriction.

Liquids.   Liquids are produced with very little obstruction in the VT, the air "flowing" around the tongue. Both [r] and [l] are voiced alveolar liquids, so the distinguishing characteristic here is tongue shape: for [l], the lateral liquid, the sides of the tongue are arched downward (lateral = side); air flows around the sides of the tongue. [r] is considered a "retroflex" liquid, because in English, the tongue is generally curled back (retro = back) during its production. Because of its retro quality, some phoneticians consider [r] to be a palatal, not alveolar, liquid.

Glides.   Glides pair up with vowels in combinations called *diphthongs*. The English glides are the velar [w] and the palatal [j], exemplified by the words *was* and *young* respectively.

Hint to Students

Older phonetics texts often used the symbol [y] for the palatal glide. The IPA has now designed [j] to represent this sound, but you may still be tempted to write [y], so be careful. See Pullum and Ladusaw (1995) and Shriberg and Kent (1995) for additional information on transcription.

Our ultimate goal is a unique "personality profile" for each speech sound as in Figure 5.1. That is, each speech sound will have a unique array of phonetic features. [d] then would be characterized as a stop consonant, [n] as a nasal consonant, [s] as a fricative consonant, and so on. We must now consider the phonetic feature of voicing.

Voicing

The state of the vocal folds is also reflected in the phonetic features of a speech sound. When the vocal folds are spread apart, and therefore still or not vibrating, voiceless sounds are produced. When the vocal folds are drawn together enough so air flow and other forces create vibration, the corresponding speech sound is voiced.

Notice on the consonant chart, Figure 5.1, that for the place for each stop and fricative—for example, bilabial stops—there are two symbols. This figure lists the voiced sound first, then the voiceless, so [b] is a voiced bilabial stop and [p] is the voiceless counterpart. Only stops, fricatives, and affricates have both voiced and voiceless speech sounds. The nasals, liquids, and glides, as well as vowels, are all voiced. We will briefly consider the voicing distinction among stop consonants measured by voice onset time (VOT).

VOT. Both [b] and [p] are bilabial stops and are distinguished further by whether the vocal folds are vibrating. They vibrate most of the time for [b], so we call that sound "voiced"; in the production of [p] the vocal folds are open and not vibrating for a relatively long portion of its production, so we consider this sound "voiceless." In the [b] consonant, the vocal folds typically begin to vibrate very quickly after the release of the consonant from the lips (short VOT), and in the "p," the vocal folds typically begin to vibrate after some delay (longer VOT). Figures 5.2 and 5.3 illustrate a voiced and voiceless initial stop, respectively, on waveforms. A waveform is a visual representation of a sound's amplitude variation across time.

While it is typical in English for voiced stops to begin with a small delay before voicing occurs, it is also possible to produce voiced stops with the voicing beginning before the release of the consonant. This results in "prevoicing" or negative VOT. Prevoicing is illustrated in Figure 5.4. Voiced stops in many languages, such as Spanish, French, and German, are typically produced with negative VOT (Ladefoged, 1993). Although English speakers sometimes do produce voiced stops with negative VOT, it is not the typical pattern. Voiced stops in English are more usually produced with either no delay between voicing onset and the release of the consonant (0 VOT) or with a short delay (short positive VOT). SLPs make use of VOT as one acoustic measure in diagnosing and treating articulatory disorders. The role of technology in aiding the SLP in such cases is discussed in chapters 9 and 17.

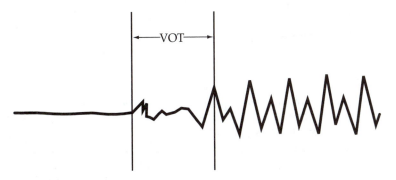

Figure 5.2 Schematic diagram of a waveform showing the voice onset time (VOT) interval for a voiced stop consonant. The left vertical line is placed at the burst onset and the right at the highest point of the first period of phonation. (Reprinted with permission by Singular Publishing Group, Inc. from J. Ryalls, *A Basic Introduction to Speech Perception*, 1996.)

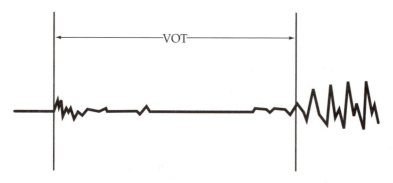

FIGURE 5.3   Schematic diagram of a waveform showing the voice onset time (VOT) interval for a voiceless stop consonant. The left vertical line is placed at the burst onset and the right at the highest point of the first period of phonation. (Reprinted with permission by Singular Publishing Group, Inc. from J. Ryalls, *A Basic Introduction to Speech Perception*, 1996).

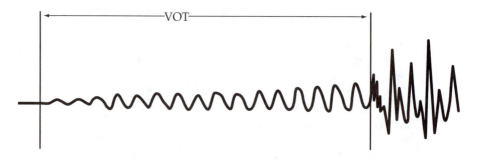

FIGURE 5.4   Schematic diagram of a waveform showing the voice onset time (VOT) interval for a prevoiced voiced stop consonant. The left vertical line is placed at the onset of phonation and the right at the burst associated with the release of the consonant. The VOT value is negative in this case, since the voicing has begun *before* the release of the consonant.

Hint to Students

You can feel an extra puff of air, called *aspiration*, when producing [p] versus [b]. In English, voiceless stops are typically produced with enough aspiration to blow out a match held in front of the speaker's lips. Voiceless stops are not produced with significant aspiration in many other languages of the world.

Vowels

The manner of articulation for vowels is characterized by an open VT and minimal obstruction of the airstream. Vowels have their own particular manner of articulation and are usually considered separately from consonants.

Vowels are characterized by the position of the tongue in the oral cavity (mouth). The tongue can be placed toward the lips or the front of the oral space, centrally placed, or back toward the velum. Likewise, the tongue can be placed higher up (toward the palate), midway down the space, or low in the mouth. A further articulatory dimension concerns whether the tongue muscles are more or less tense or relaxed (lax). Finally, we need to know if the lips are rounded or not (rounding). The articulatory dimensions we discussed that define vowels, then, are front-back, high-low, tense-lax, and the presence or absence of rounding.

All vowels are voiced (unless they are whispered), and the place of articulation feature is replaced by the dimensions of tongue position around the oral cavity.

Vowels are often represented in a schematic chart called the *vowel space*, representing the oral cavity as in Figure 5.5. Think of a side view of a speaker facing to the left. The upper left cell, then, would be the tongue at its highest and most front position. The vowel sound produced in this position is the vowel sound in the word *see*, and it is represented as [i] in the International Phonetic Alphabet. The highest and most back sound in the vowel space is [u], as in *Sue*. The other dimensions and accompanying symbols, with English examples, are shown below. Note that this correspondence between tongue position and phonetic feature is a simplification. Not all speakers produce [i] higher than [e], for example (Peterson & Barney, 1952).

Hint to Students

The vowel space is sometimes called the vowel quadrangle. In Figure 5.5, it is depicted as a triangle. Because the oral cavity narrows towards the back, such shapes depict the vowel space better than would a square.

Unlike the features of consonants, vowel features are not necessarily binary, although the use of pluses and minuses remains. [ɑ], as in *pot*, for example, is a [+low] vowel, but [−low] does not necessarily mean [+high], for it can also mean the tongue is midway down the oral cavity.

Notice that in the front column there are five symbols. In our quest for unique descriptions of speech sounds, we would need to distinguish further between the high vowels, the low vowels, and so on. Tension in the tongue muscles is one distinction that is used. The slightly higher vowel is considered [+tense], the lower counterpart being [−tense], or more commonly as [+lax].

Hint to Students

In general, English syllables may end in a tense vowel but not a lax one. We have the word [si], for example, but [sI] would be non-English. Vowels such as [æ] and [ɑ] can be identified as tense or lax by testing if they can end an English syllable. [mɑ] is allowed, but [mæ] would not be allowed. So [ɑ] is considered a tense vowel, and [æ] is lax.]

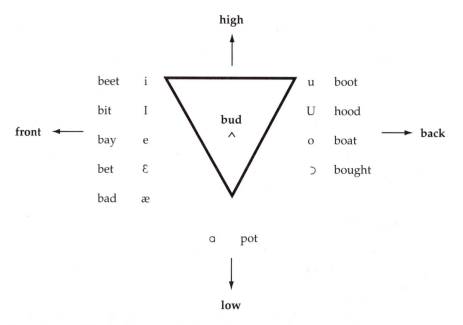

FIGURE 5.5   Schematic representation of some vowels of American English arranged according to tongue placement. (Reprinted with permission by Singular Publishing Group, Inc. from J. Ryalls, *A Basic Introduction to Speech Perception*, 1996).

Finally, in the center of the vowel space is the wedge (or caret). This vowel sound can be heard in monosyllabic, stressed words such as *but* and *cup*. The unstressed version of this vowel is the schwa vowel [ə] (which does not appear in Figure 5.5). Their distinction is not one of tense versus lax features, but instead where in a word's stress pattern they occur. The schwa occurs in unstressed syllables, as in the final syllable of *sofa* or the initial syllable of *about*. Remember that the wedge occurs in stressed syllables, as in monosyllables such as *cut* and *putt*.

Hint to Students

It is to your benefit to memorize both the consonant and vowel charts, Figures 5.1 and 5.5. You may resist at first, but by internalizing the place-manner-voicing features of the consonants and phonetic features of vowels, your understanding of speech production is advanced tremendously.

Acoustic Phonetics

Acoustically, speech sounds are all complex sounds in that they are composed of more than one single frequency value. Artificial speech created on a computer with only a single pure tone sounds robotic and is difficult to perceive as speech without being primed for it. Figure 5.6 depicts a pure tone and a complex tone. The axes used to describe these sounds show a sound's amplitude across time.

Hint to Students

Due to the human vocal anatomy, speech is never pure in tone—it is complex.

This depiction of speech is called a *waveform*. In Figure 5.6A, the *pure tone*, the waveform takes on a sinusoidal shape, repeating in a regularly spaced fashion. This picture of speech shows a single frequency component—only a single frequency value—so vibration is unchanging at every point along the time axis. Figure 5.6B, also a waveform, shows a *complex tone* comprised of more than one frequency component.

Hint to Students

A regular but non-sinusoidal waveform with a variety of peaks is a depiction of a complex sound.

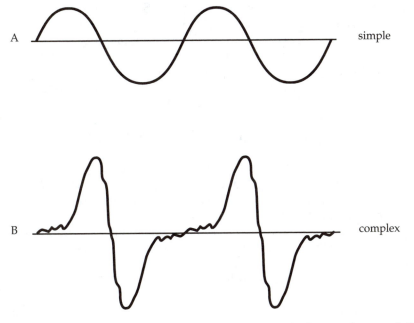

FIGURE 5.6   Schematic diagram of (A) a simple periodic waveform, and (B) a complex periodic waveform.

From a waveform alone, we cannot tell how many components make up a complex sound or what frequency they are. Other measures are more appropriate for complex tones.

Speech sounds fall into two additional categories, *periodic* and *aperiodic*, depending on the path the air from the lungs takes through the vocal folds and out the vocal tract. The vocal folds are considered the sound source and the vocal tract the filter for the sound. This theory of speech production is called the *source-filter theory* (Lieberman & Blumstein, 1988). A typical periodic speech sound contains a repeating pattern; that is, there is a regularity to the acoustic waveform as it comes out from the lips. Any voiced sound is periodic since there is a regular alternation of the airstream at the glottis. In other words, the vocal folds impact regularity, and hence periodicity, to a speech sound. This periodicity is known as the *fundamental frequency*.

Constriction in the vocal tract, if sufficient, causes some noise-like irregularity in the sound. The vocal tract is then considered a sound source, since it generates a noise sound source. Therefore, consonants with a great deal of constriction (stops, fricatives, affricatives) would be considered aperiodic sounds since they have an aperiodic sound source. The voiced stops, fricatives and affricates, which change from one sound source to another, would therefore be considered both aperiodic and periodic. Vowels, nasals, glides, and liquids, which are voiced and produced with little constriction, are all periodic sounds. Again, while nasals are produced with oral constriction, the air flows freely through the nasal cavity. Hence the nasal consonants are periodic.

We said earlier that the rate at which a speaker's vocal folds vibrate is the fundamental frequency for that speaker. Speech, however, does not have acoustic energy simply at the fundamental frequency (hereafter, abbreviated f_o). Due to various properties of the vocal folds, not only does energy exist at the f_o, but also at whole number multiples of the f_o. These whole number multiples of the fundamental are known as *harmonics*. An adult male with an f_o of 100 Hertz (or cycles per second, hereafter abbreviate Hz) will have energy at 100 Hz, but also at 100×2 or 200 Hz, 100×3 or 300 Hz, 100×4 or 400 Hz, and so on in decreasing amplitude. These harmonics are also the product of vocal fold vibration. The f_o is technically considered the first harmonic (1 times any number equals that number).

These same calculations can be made for different f_o values. An adult female speaker's f_o may be 200 Hz. Notice that the second harmonic is 200×2 or 400 Hz. The third harmonic is 200×3 or 600 Hz. The fourth harmonic is 200×4 or 800 Hz. It is important to note that the value of the f_o is also the interval between harmonics. In other words, since harmonics are whole-number multiples of the f_o, the space between them will be this same base value, and the harmonics will be evenly spaced across the frequency range.

Harmonics tend to steadily drop off in amplitude at higher and higher frequencies. For speech, there is typically a 12 dB (decibels, a unit of amplitude) reduction in amplitude for each doubling of the f_o. A doubling of the f_o is also

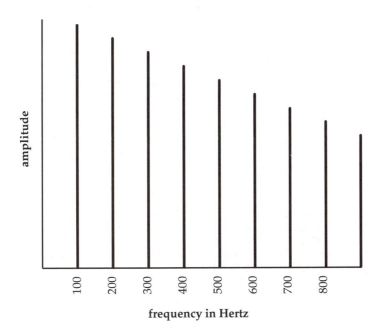

FIGURE 5.7 **Diagram of a source spectrum for a voice with a fundamental frequency of 100 Hertz.**

known as one *octave*. This drop-off in amplitude is called *damping*—the loss of amplitude at higher frequencies (see Figure 5.7). Notice that the X-axes on these measures are in frequency and not in time like those of a waveform. These are called *spectra* (plural of a single *spectrum*). Spectra are better representations of complex sounds, because they record individual frequency values.

To return to vowel sounds, when the tongue is placed in a certain position in the mouth, the oral cavity is divided into two chambers—one in front of the tongue and the other in back of the tongue and extending down to the vocal folds. When the vocal folds are vibrating, the sound is then modified by these two chambers. The way in which the sound of the vocal folds is modified is known as *resonance*, which will be considered in more detail in the next chapter.

Format frequencies, the frequency values amplified due to the configuration of the VT, are the acoustic correlates that determine a vowel. Since consonants are produced with very rapid movements of the articulators, the acoustic information that results is also very rapidly changing. In fact, there is some debate as to which acoustic information uniquely specifies consonants. We are now ready to consider the role that the VT plays in the production of speech. In the next chapter, we examine this aspect of speech production called resonance.

Study Questions

1. What is the purpose of the IPA?

2. What are phonetic features?

3. What is the difference between place and manner of articulation?

4. In what ways are vowels different from consonants?

5. What are two ways to visually present speech? What are the advantages of each?

References

Ladefoged, P. (1993). *A course in phonetics* (3rd ed.). Fort Worth, TX: Harcourt Brace Jovanovich.

Lieberman, P., & Blumstein, S. (1988). *Speech physiology, speech perception, and acoustic phonetics.* New York: Cambridge University Press.

Peterson, G., & Barney, H. (1952). Control methods used in a study of the vowels. *Journal of the Acoustical Society of America, 24,* 175–184.

Pullum, G., & Ladusaw, W. (1995). *Phonetic symbol guide* (2nd ed.). Chicago: University of Chicago Press.

Shriberg, L., & Kent, R. (1995). *Clinical phonetics* (2nd ed.). Boston: Allyn & Bacon.

CHAPTER

6

Resonance

While *articulation* refers to movements of the tongue and other articulators (such as the lips) in producing speech, *resonance* refers to the acoustic response of the supralaryngeal vocal tract. Remember that the supralaryngeal vocal tract refers to the structures above the vocal folds and includes three resonating spaces or cavities: (1) the oral (i.e., mouth) cavity, (2) the nasal (i.e., nose) cavity, and (3) the pharyngeal (i.e., throat) cavity. When the vocal folds are vibrating in phonation, this sound is modified or "filtered" by the vocal tract. That is why this account of speech production is known as the source-filter theory of speech production. The vibrating vocal folds provide a sound source, which is then filtered by the vocal tract.

Although the actual vocal tract is curved or bent at almost 90 degrees in human beings, many of the acoustic properties of the vocal tract can be understood in terms of a single resonating tube. Thus, we will begin our discussion of vocal tract resonance in terms of one single resonating tube or chamber.

Basic Properties of Resonance

In order to understand vocal tract resonance, we first have to comprehend some of the basic properties of resonance. To get at some of these basic properties, let's begin with the simple metaphor of a soft drink bottle. We all know that a soft drink bottle will whistle or resonate a certain sound when air is blown across the top of the bottle at just the right angle. Most of us also realize that the sound that this bottle will produce depends on how much liquid is in the bottle. When the bottle is empty, the tone that is produced is fairly deep or low. As the bottle is filled with more and more liquid, the resonating sound gets higher and higher in pitch because the resonating air space gets progressively smaller. Put differently, when filling a container with liquid, the pitch of the sound created by pouring in the liquid gets higher as the liquid gets nearer to the top of the container. From these analogies, then, we can learn two important properties about vocal tract resonance: (1) that air blown through, or into, a hollow chamber (actually filled with air particles) in a certain manner can cause the chamber to vibrate or resonate at a certain frequency; and (2) the smaller the resonating chamber, the higher the resonating frequency.

From our discussion of phonation and the fundamental frequency, you will recall that a complex periodic wave not only has energy present at its basic or fundamental frequency, but also has energy at whole number multiples or harmonics of this fundamental. In fact, resonance affects these harmonics. That is, some harmonics are emphasized and others are suppressed or *dampened*. The result of resonance is that the shape of the harmonic spectrum is changed. Instead of falling off in an orderly even manner, peaks and valleys are created. The peaks of this harmonic spectrum, which has been filtered by the vocal tract, are known as *formants*.

Figure 6.1 depicts the change in the source spectrum after it has been filtered by the vocal tract. The peaks in the speech output spectrum on the right of the diagram are the formants.

Although we also hear the fundamental frequency of a speaker's voice, formant frequencies are the most important frequency characteristics of speech. Formant frequencies are the acoustic properties that distinguish the various vowels. Figure 6.2 shows a linear predictive coding spectrum of an /i/ vowel. Linear predictive coding, or LPC, is a mathematical procedure that locates formant frequencies. The first three formant peaks are labeled F_1, F_2, and F_3 respectively, and their corresponding frequency values are given at the right of the figure.

Right away, it is important to point out that formants are very different from the harmonics of the fundamental frequency. While harmonics are whole number multiples of the f_0, formant frequencies do not bear any predictable mathematical relationship with the f_0. Harmonics and formants are easy for students to confuse because they both relate to speech and they are both measured in Hertz (or cycles per second). However, formants do not bear a direct relationship to the f_0. We cannot tell a thing about formants from knowing the f_0. Rather, it is necessary to have some idea of the position of the tongue. But even when we know the tongue's position, we cannot predict formant frequencies very well. Tongue position can give us some information about likely formant frequencies, but f_0, or the rate of vibration of the vocal folds, is completely independent from the formant frequencies.

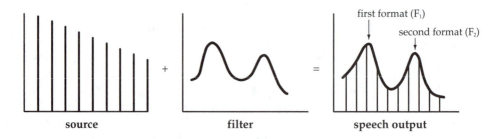

FIGURE 6.1   Diagram of the filtering effects of the vocal tract. A source spectrum is filtered by the vocal tract to result in a speech output spectrum—in this case a vowel. The first formant (F_1) and second formant (F_2) are labeled in the vowel output spectrum.

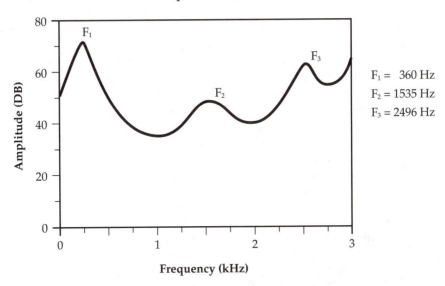

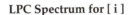

LPC Spectrum for [i]

$F_1 = 360$ Hz
$F_2 = 1535$ Hz
$F_3 = 2496$ Hz

FIGURE 6.2   Linear predictive coding (LPC) spectrum for an /i/ vowel produced by an adult male speaker and measured on the BLISS speech analysis system. Formants 1, 2 and 3 are labeled and the frequency values are printed at the right of the figure. See text for details. (Reprinted with permission by Singular Publishing Group, Inc. from J. Ryalls, *A Basic Introduction to Speech Perception*, 1996)

Hint to Students

Harmonics are the fundamental frequency (f_o) and all multiples of the fundamental; they are products of the vocal folds. Formants are labeled F_1, F_2, and so on, but they are products of the vocal tract. Do not confuse F_1 for a harmonic or f_o for a formant frequency.

How do we know that harmonics and formants are independent? It is this independence of fundamental frequency and formant frequencies that allows us to sing. In singing, we are varying the fundamental frequency (which we hear as pitch) of our voices, while employing the formant frequencies to deliver the lyrics or words of the song. If formant frequencies were dependent upon the fundamental frequency, then changing the notes of a song would also change the words! To keep these two separate, think of the following. An individual can produce the same vowel with different fundamental frequencies, or inversely, that individual can produce different vowels with the same fundamental frequency. Therefore, the two are separate. It is the independence of the two that makes speech so communicatively rich.

Of course, two people can have different fundamental frequencies, producing the same vowel such as [i]. In this case, the formants and the fundamental frequency will *both* be different (although the frequency difference between the first two formants for [i] remains the similar).

Although for most vowels it is almost impossible to predict formant frequencies simply from knowing tongue position, there is one vowel where it is possible to predict formant frequencies without knowing detailed information about tongue position. This is the case of the neutral or schwa vowel, [ə] (the unstressed version of the wedge [^]). Because the tongue is lying along the floor of the mouth for this vowel, the tongue does not affect vocal tract resonance to any significant degree. While for most of the vowels, the tongue divides the vocal tract into two resonating chambers (one in front of the tongue, and one in back of the tongue), for schwa the vocal tract is essentially a single tube extending from the lips down to the vocal folds. Of course, there is a right-angle bend in the tube, but otherwise the vocal tract is essentially a tube that is open at one end (at the lips) and closed at the other (the larynx). In the schwa vowel, the spaces in front and in back of the tongue are more or less equal. That is, the oral and pharyngeal cavities are approximately equal in size.

A tube that is open at one end and closed at the other has some special properties. Such a tube is known as a *quarter-wave resonator* because its lowest resonant frequency is a quarter the length of the tube. There is a scientific formula that will allow us to predict the formant frequencies of this tube that is open at one end and closed at the other. This formula is: Frequency in Hertz = the speed of sound (SS) divided by 4 times the length of the tube (l). This gives us the formula $F = SS/4 \times l$. Although there are different ways to estimate these formants, we will use the values given by Kent (1997). The typical length of the adult male vocal tract is about 17.5 centimeters. Knowing that the speed of sound is a constant 350 meters per second, we can solve the equation. First of all, we have to change the length of the adult male vocal tract into meters since it is in centimeters. To do so, we have to divide by 100 (centimeters = 1/100 of a meter). This gives us .175 meters. 350 divided by 4 × .175 meters = 350 divided by .7 = 500. We would come up with approximately 500 Hz for the lowest resonant frequency.

Having calculated 500 Hz for the lowest resonant frequency or formant, there is another special property of the quarter-wave resonator that will allow us to predict the next two formant frequencies. That is, a quarter-wave resonator only reinforces odd multiples. In other words, unlike harmonics in which every multiple of the fundamental frequency is emphasized, in a quarter-wave resonator only odd-numbered multiples of the lowest resonant frequency are emphasized.

Counting off the odd numbers from 1 to 5, the first one we arrive at is, of course, the number 1, and 1 × 1 = 1. We have already discovered that the lowest resonant frequency is approximately 500 Hz. The next number we come across is 2, but 2 is an even number so it is not used. The next number is 3, and it is an odd number so we use it: 3 × 500 Hz = 1500 Hz, which is the next resonant frequency or the approximate second formant frequency for schwa. The next number after 3 is 4. But 4 is another even number, so it drops out. The next number is 5, which is an odd number again, so we use it: 5 × 500 Hz = 2500 Hz.

So, knowing the approximate length of the vocal tract and the speed of sound, along with the special properties of the quarter-wave resonator, we can approximate that the first three formant frequencies of schwa produced by an adult male are 500 Hz, 1500 Hz, and 2500 Hz respectively. Now of course, these are approximations. You may not find that acoustic studies give formant frequencies for schwa that correspond to these values. Since the real world is also composed of women and children, we consider these speakers as well. Approximate values for F1 and F2 for a schwa vowel produced by a woman or a child would be higher because their vocal tracts are smaller and thus their resonating cavities are smaller, which leads to higher formant values.

Once again, schwa is the only vowel for which it is possible to predict something about formant frequencies without knowing the position of the tongue. This is because the tongue is not much in the way, and the vocal tract is approximately one single resonating tube. It is also not possible to predict formant frequencies for the other vowels in such a direct and simple manner. In fact, we will not attempt to do so because mathematical modeling of these acoustic events is much too complex for an introductory text on speech science. However, even though we will not attempt to predict exact formant frequency values on the basis of tongue position, we will point out some general relative properties of formant frequencies, based on the position of the tongue. There is research showing that the articulatory positions denoted in the IPA do not hold for every speaker. That is, some speakers produce [e] with a higher tongue position than [i]. This is why we will only point out relative positions.

Basic Properties of Formant Frequencies

Before we discuss general properties of formant frequencies, it is important to emphasize that what we are about to discuss is a drastic simplification. Formant frequencies are not so directly related to size of the resonating chambers within the vocal tract. However, this simplification will serve the purposes of most beginning SLPs and audiologists. Students who learn about predicting formant frequencies from tongue position and shape of the vocal tract in this simplified manner may encounter a somewhat more accurate and more complicated model at a later point in time. Remember, what you have learned about the relationship between tongue position and formant frequency values is a simplification. Bearing this in mind, the following principle will allow students to understand the basic associations behind tongue position and formant frequencies.

In simple terms, the size and shape of the back cavity is associated with the frequency value of F_1, and the size and shape of the front (oral) cavity is associated with the F_2 value. In the vowel /i/ (as in *bee*) the tongue is in its highest, most front position. Since the tongue is high and front in the mouth, the resonating chamber in front of the tongue is small, so the frequency at which this chamber resonates is relatively high.

Hint to Students

F_1 is generally associated with the space behind the tongue or pharyngeal cavity; F_2 is generally associated with the space in front of the tongue or oral cavity.

In fact, since this vowel has the highest tongue position, it also has the smallest oral cavity and the highest second formant frequency. Compared to /i/, all the other vowels have a lower second formant (or F_2). Since the tongue is high and front in the mouth, the chamber in back of the tongue is relatively large. We know that relatively large resonating chambers resonate at relatively low frequencies. For the vowel /i/, F_1 is very low, F_2 relatively high. In fact, /i/ is the vowel with the greatest difference between F_1 and F_2.

As the tongue moves back from this high front position, in general, the oral cavity becomes larger and F_2 consequently becomes lower in frequency. Likewise, the pharyngeal cavity behind the tongue becomes smaller and consequently F_1 becomes higher. In a very general manner, then, as the vowels proceed from the highest, most front vowel—/i/ to /I/ to /ɛ/ to /e/ to /æ/, and then up the back series from /ɔ/ to /o/ to /ʊ/ to /u/—the distance between the two formants is successively reduced. The complicating factor is lip rounding in the non-low back vowels of English. Protruding the lips extends the general length of the vocal tract, thereby lowering both formant frequencies.

Table 6.1 gives average F_1, F_2, and F_3 values from a group of adult male, adult female, and child speakers for the vowels /i/,/ɑ/, and /u/ from a study by Peterson and Barney (1952). Notice again how a large cavity is associated with a low formant value, while a small cavity is associated with a higher formant value. With rounded vowels, such as [u], lip protrusion acts to lengthen the oral cavity and thus also lowers the F_2 value. Notice that F_3 values do not vary as greatly as the first two formants between the different vowels.

TABLE 6.1   Average Formant Frequency Values in Hertz

		/i/	/ɑ/	/u/
Adult Males	F_1	270	730	300
	F_2	2290	1090	870
	F_3	3010	2440	2240
Adult Females	F_1	310	850	370
	F_2	2790	1220	950
	F_3	3310	2810	2670
Children	F_1	370	1030	430
	F_2	3200	1370	1170
	F_3	3730	3170	3260

Source: Adapted from Peterson & Barney (1952).

The simple association of a formant value with a resonating cavity gives us a basic understanding of the contribution of vocal tract resonance to the vowels and demonstrates a direct link between articulation and the acoustic properties of speech sounds. While formants account for vowels in a rather direct manner, formant frequencies do not explain consonants in so direct a fashion.

In other words, while it is difficult to predict the formant frequencies of vowels other than schwa, it is even harder to predict the formant pattern for consonants, which can be both periodic and aperiodic. We will briefly review the consonants, first of all considering the manner of articulation.

Consonants

Stops

Stop production, you will remember, is characterized by complete closure somewhere in the oral cavity, a build-up of air pressure behind that closure, and a sudden release of the closure resulting in a burst of air. Because of this small "explosion" of air, stops are also sometimes called *plosives*. Acoustically, the stop burst is an aperiodic spike of energy followed by the onset of voicing for any subsequent speech sound. Voiced and voiceless stops are largely differentiated by voice onset time (VOT, see chapter 5). Voiceless stops are also associated with bursts of higher amplitude than are voiced stops.

Technically, stops cannot be isolated from other speech sounds in a syllable. Experimenters have attempted to present listeners with just the burst or a short segment of burst and a following vowel; listeners consistently respond that they hear the whole syllable, or a nonspeech sound (Liberman, Cooper, Shankweiler, & Studdert-Kennedy, 1967). The vocal tract changes quickly from the release of closure to subsequent speech sounds, so the formants will show sudden change as well. These changes are called *formant transitions* and can be contrasted with the more horizontal, steady-state formant for speech sounds such as vowels. See Figure 6.3 for the difference between the steady-state portion and the transition portion of a formant.

Nasals

Nasal consonants make use of the nasal cavity, which lengthens the vocal tract as a whole and suppresses energy. This third cavity also adds some low-frequency nasal murmuring to the acoustic nature of [m], [n], and [ŋ].

Fricatives

The narrow passage in the vocal tract created by articulators approaching but not making contact creates turbulence (friction) in the airstream. Acoustically, fricatives show a great deal of aperiodic energy in waveforms, with voiced fricatives showing a more regular pattern due to the regularity of vocal fold vibration.

transition | steady state

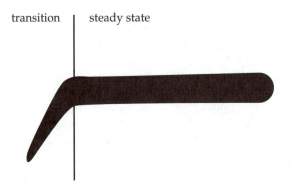

FIGURE 6.3   Schematic diagram of a formant frequency with the transition and steady- state portions labeled. (Reprinted with permission by Singular Publishing Group, Inc. from J. Ryalls, *A Basic Introduction to Speech Perception*, 1996)

Affricates

The acoustic properties of the stop and fricative components of affricates can be seen in waveforms. A burst (release of closure) is apparent, but instead of a sudden transition to the following speech sound, affricates gradually move into the articulatory position for a fricative.

Liquids and Glides

These sounds have relatively little vocal tract constriction and are considered periodic consonants. Their formants have very long, gradual transitions to the following sounds. Although their formant transitions are relatively long, they are not as long, however, as those for diphthong vowels. One can distinguish among the liquid and glide sounds by measuring the F_2 and F_3 values. [w] and [j] have very extreme F_2 values, the [w] associated with the very low F_2 of [u] and [j] the very high F_2 of [l]. The F_2 for liquids falls intermediately between these values. One can distinguish [r] from [l] acoustically by the F_3 value: [r] has a low F_3 while [l] is associated with a high value. This F_3 distinction is due to the tongue shape for each liquid: lateral for [l] and retroflex for [r].

In the next chapter, we take a look at how speech sounds combine to form words. We will discuss phonology, the study of sound patterns in a language.

Study Questions

1. Explain the difference between formant frequencies and harmonics.

2. How do the following articulatory maneuvers affect the value of formants:

Rounding the lips?

Raising the tongue?

Fronting the tongue?

3. What is the acoustic distinction between a voiced consonant and a voiceless consonant?

References

Kent, R. (1997). *The speech sciences*. San Diego, CA: Singular Publishing Group.

Liberman, A., Cooper, F., Shankweiler, D., & Studdert-Kennedy, M. (1967). Perception of the speech code. *Psychological Review, 74,* 431–461.

Peterson, G., & Barney, H. (1952). Control methods used in a study of the vowels. *Journal of the Acoustical Society of America, 24,* 175–184.

CHAPTER

7

Phonology

We have already discussed phonetics, the study of speech sounds. In this chapter, we will investigate phonology. *Phonology* is the study of sound patterns, how speech sounds influence one another when arranged into words. When a speaker sequences consonants and vowels into syllables and words, the arrangement of segments may influence the articulatory and acoustic properties of sounds.

Importance of Phonology

Phonology is one of the levels of linguistic knowledge acquired as one develops a native language system. Phonology is of concern to SLPs who are diagnosing and treating clients with both speech impairments and language disorders. Clinicians need to be aware of deficiencies that may arise at the level of phonological processing. Concentrating only on impairments at the level of the individual speech sound may cause an SLP to miss the larger picture of sound combinations and word contexts. A speaker may have trouble with production of voiceless fricatives, for example, but only when they occur between two vowels (i.e., intervocalically).

Speech sounds in isolation can be described by phonetic features. [æ], for example, is a low, front, unrounded vowel. Such a feature description, however, is basically an ideal, an abstraction. Remember that when speech sound segments are combined into syllables and words, they may influence neighboring segments. In addition, languages allow certain combinations of segments and block other combinations, an area of study known as *phonotactics*.

Let's look at an example of a speech sound altered by a neighboring segment. Vowels in English are non-nasal (oral), reflecting the fact that during production the nasal cavity is closed. However, when a vowel is followed by a nasal consonant, as in the word *can*, American English speakers will anticipate the upcoming nasal consonant while still producing the vowel, and thus open the nasal cavity early, during vowel production. The result is that most American speakers produce a nasal quality on any vowel preceding a nasal segment (Keefe & Dalton, 1989).

Writing Speech Sounds

Phonology differentiates between an abstract version of a speech sound and the realized speech sound as actually produced. At the level of abstraction, these ideal speech sounds are called *phonemes*. They are written in the IPA using slash marks to set them off. Thus, an English vowel at the phonemic level of abstraction would be non-nasal and represented as /a/, /æ/, or /ɪ/. To represent any vowel, a capital V cover-symbol is frequently used in phonology. We can say, then, that phonemically, English vowels are /V/.

When a speech sound is produced, it may not have exactly the same phonetic features as the original phoneme. Remember that /V/ is actually realized as nasalized in a certain context: preceding a nasal consonant. When produced, that phoneme is represented with square brackets, not slash marks, and the spoken version of the abstract phoneme is called a *phone*. The phoneme /æ/ in the word *can*, then, is written as the nasalized phone [æ̃]. When realized at the phonetic level, a speech sound is not represented by slash marks (//) around the IPA symbol, but rather by square brackets ([]). The tilde (~) over the IPA symbol represents nasal quality and is called a *diacritic*. A diacritic is a symbol showing an alteration in sound quality when a phoneme is produced.

/æ/ of course can also be produced without nasal quality in words such as *cat* and *bat*, where no nasal consonant is around to add nasality to a neighboring vowel. In these cases, the phoneme /æ/ is realized as the phone [æ]. What we have, then, is a case where a single phoneme (an abstract ideal) is realized in two different ways: nasalized and unnasalized.

Hint to Students

Phonemes are never actually spoken. They are ideals, uninfluenced by context. Spoken sounds are called phones. Phonemes are represented with slash marks, phones with square brackets. Orthography, the spelling of a word, is usually noted by italics to show that it is a word and not a sequence of phonetic symbols.

At the phonemic level, a word like *can* starts out as a series of phonemes— /k/ /æ/ /n/—combined without contextual influence as /k æ n/. In actual production by an American English speaker, this sequence of speech sounds changes phonetic features in a predictable way; it is represented phonetically as [k æ̃ n]. Compare it to a word like *cat*, which is represented phonemically as /k æ t/ and phonetically as [k æ t], without vowel nasalization.

You may wonder why we would bother with two levels of representation for a word like *cat* if both representations look the same. That is just a coincidence in this case. Often, the phonemic and phonetic levels differ, and we need to signal what level we are discussing. SLPs also would need to clarify what level of phonology they are describing and dealing with when working with a client: the underlying phonemic representation, or the spoken phonetic level. Either or both levels may be impaired in a particular client (see discussion on aphasia in chapters 13 and 16).

Additional Concepts

We now need to add some additional terminology. Notice that the term "phone" denotes any spoken, realized speech sound, but that the term does not signal what phoneme underlies the sound. All phones derive from some phoneme, and phonology is concerned with the relationship between phonemes and phones in a language. [æ] and [æ̃] derive from the same underlying phoneme: /æ/. In a sense, they are the same speech sound in a language user's mind. This is not necessarily true for languages other than English. French, for example, has nasalized vowels at the phonemic level (Schane, 1968). Phonologists need to consider each language separately to determine the relationship between phones and phonemes. If one were to nasalize the vowel in *cat* or denasalize the vowel in *can*, these words would not change their meaning, although these productions might sound unusual to native speakers (Fromkin & Rodman, 1998).

Allophones

In English, [æ] and [æ̃] are *allophones* of the same phoneme: They derive from the same phoneme and the feature by which they differ is not very important to the phonology, at least for speakers of English. If speakers were to add nasalization to, or delete it from, an English vowel, they would not be altering the meaning of words. We can say that the difference between two allophones of the same phoneme is linguistically nondistinctive, or that the feature in question (here nasality on vowels) is not linguistically distinctive.

Hint to Students

Not all allophones of the same phoneme are always represented with the same IPA symbol plus diacritic on one allophone. [r] and [l], for example, are allophones of the phoneme /l/ in Korean (Fromkin & Rodman, 1998).

Coarticulation

Phonological changes due to the ordering of segments often can be traced to human anatomy and articulation. In the case of [kæ̃n], the addition of nasality on the vowel is due to a phonological process called *coarticulation*. While producing one phone, the articulators are simultaneously moving for a second phone. Thus, an American English speaker would be producing a vowel and the nasality of the nasal consonant simultaneously in *can* or in any other word with a vowel followed immediately by a nasal consonant.

Notice that opening the nasal cavity does not interfere with the articulation needed to produce a vowel, that is, tongue placement in the oral cavity and, perhaps, lip rounding. For French vowels, nasality is a distinctive feature, so speakers of French would only produce nasalized vowels when the phoneme underlying the phone is nasalized.

We can predict when a vowel will be nasalized in English, since nasality on vowels is not distinctive in English (this is not true for French). A certain context or word environment "causes" the vowel to nasalize; we say the environment conditions the change in sound quality. A vowel immediately preceding a nasal consonant will predictably be nasalized in American English. This process can be described with a system of symbols in a logical, cause and effect manner as /V/ → +nasal/____N. This "phonological rule" can be read as follows: "Any phonemic vowel is realized as a nasalized phone when it occurs in the environment immediately preceding a nasal consonant." The arrow denotes a change when one speaks and produces a sound. The slash can be read as "in the environment of," and the blank slot would be the placement of the speech sound in question used in a particular word. The N is our cover symbol for any nasal consonant.

We can now expand this rule to include the unnasalized phone of the vowel, which occurs in all places *except* before N. We would call those environments "everywhere else" or "elsewhere."

$$/V/ \rightarrow +nasal/\underline{\quad}N$$
$$\rightarrow -nasal/ \text{ elsewhere}$$

Given this rule, our phonological system looks for vowels placed before nasal consonants and nasalizes them. All other vowels maintain their [–nasal] feature.

Unfortunately, it would be an oversimplification to state that nasalization in English is linguistically nondistinct. That statement would only be true for vowels. Nasality in consonants is a different story. Take [b] and [m]. These are two phones in English. They differ, feature-wise, in exactly the same way that [æ] and [æ̃] differ: one is +nasal and one is –nasal. You may resist this argument. After all, [æ] and [æ̃] are basically the same phonetic symbol of IPA with a diacritic showing a nondistinctive difference. [m] and [b] are two separate symbols in IPA and of the English alphabet. But let's examine the phonetic feature profiles for the sounds in question in Table 7.1.

Each pair differs by only one feature, nasality. If you are still resisting this line of reasoning, you may be sensing a different level of importance to the [+nasal] feature for a consonant compared to a vowel. And you would be correct!

Remember that nasalization on a vowel does not change what phoneme it stems from, nor would it alter word meaning if added to a non-nasalized vowel.

TABLE 7.1 Phonetic Feature Profiles

[æ]	[æ̃]	[b]	[m]
+front	+front	+bilabial	+bilabial
+low	+low	+voiced	+voiced
–nasal	+nasal	–nasal	+nasal

Nasality on vowels is phonologically nondistinctive. Nasality on consonants, however, *is* phonologically distinctive. Adding or deleting nasality on a consonant would alter the phonemic level of the sound and change the meaning of a word with that sound segment in it: *bat* plus nasality on the [b] gives *mat*, a different word; *bat* plus nasality on the [æ] vowel still gives *bat*, just pronounced with a nasal vowel ("nasal twang") instead.

[b] and [m] are not allophones of the same phoneme the way [æ] and [æ̃] are. They are two separate phonemes. [b] derives from the phoneme /b/ and [m] derives from the phoneme /m/. In these cases, each phoneme is realized as only one allophone and can be written by the following rules:

$$/b/ \rightarrow [b] / \text{ everywhere}$$
$$/m/ \rightarrow [m] / \text{ everywhere}$$

Hint to Students

Allophonic variation of consonantal phonemes in English does occur. For example, there is a nondistinctive variation of the amount of air produced with a voiceless stop, depending on where in a word the stop occurs. Word-initially, voiceless stops are associated with more air release than stops word-medially or finally. The amount of air released with the stop does not alter the meaning of the word in which the phone occurs.

Minimal Pairs

Words that "test" whether two phones are allophones of the same phoneme or derive from separate phonemes are called *minimal pairs*. A minimal pair is a set of words that differs in only one way and shifts meaning due to that linguistic difference. [b æ t] and [m æ t] compose a minimal pair: They differ in one way, the presence or absence of nasality on the initial consonant. They change meaning depending on the presence or absence of that feature.

In contrast, there is no minimal pair in English that differs by only the presence or absence of nasality on a vowel. If one can find a minimal pair (such as [b æ t] and [m æ t]), the feature difference is distinctive and those two different segments are from separate phonemes. When no minimal pair can be found for a feature difference, those two phones are allophones of the same phoneme and the feature is not linguistically distinctive.

Hint to Students

When no minimal pair exists for the two segments, those speech sounds are allophones of the same phoneme. In other words, the feature in question is linguistically nondistinctive. The presence or abscence of those speech sounds (and that feature) is predictable.

The placement of nasality on consonants cannot be predicted. Consider the following environment : #___æ t. This collection of symbols represents a specific position in a word and can be read as follows: a speech sound at the beginning of a word and followed by the segments [æ] and [t]. # is a symbol for a word boundary, either the beginning or end of a word. Here it designates the word beginning.

Could you predict if [b] or [m] would occur in this word position? No, because either phone could. A nasal or non-nasal consonant could appear word-initially and be followed by [æ t]: [b æ t] or [m æ t]. In contrast, you can always predict where a nasalized vowel will occur—before a nasal consonant.

Hint to Students

The existence of a minimal pair means the feature in question is phonologically distinctive; the alternating segments are allophones of separate phonemes. The occurrence of the feature in question cannot be predicted.

Implications for Speech Therapy

Speech-language pathologists need to understand the way speech sounds are phonemically represented in speakers' minds in order to know if a production impairment is at the phonetic level or the phonemic level. In other words, is the mistake in language or in articulation of the word? Would a production problem impair comprehension of a word? Saying *mat* for *bat* would be a more serious error than producing *cat* with a nasalized vowel.

Coarticulation may be another focus of speech therapy. Remember that coarticulation is a phonetic process whereby more than one articulatory maneuver is associated with the production of a speech sound, due to contextual influence. There are actually two types of coarticulation: *anticipatory* and *carryover* (Ladefoged, 1993). In anticipatory coarticulation (also called right to left coarticulation), a speech sound is influenced by a following segment. So a vowel being nasalized by a following nasal consonant is an example of anticipating the nasal, and hence anticipatory coarticulation. The feature spreads from right to left.

Another example of anticipatory coarticulation involves consonant change. Take the two words *key* and *coo*. The placement of /k/ before the front vowel /i/ in the first word is more toward the hard palate, while /k/ produced before the back vowel /u/ in *coo* is produced closer to the velum. Tongue placement for /k/, then, is influenced by the phonetic feature (articulation) of the following vowel, a right-to-left influence. Notice, though, that the fronting of /k/ doesn't actually result in a different phone, such as the alveolar stop /t/.

Carryover (or left to right) coarticulation may also occur in speech. A phonetic feature of a segment carries over and influences the following segment. For example, consider the two words *beat* and *boot*. While word-final /t/ in both words is phonemically the same, /t/ in *boot* is pronounced with more lip-rounding than is /t/ in *beat*. The property of the rounded vowel has spread to the following consonant. (Actually, this is an example of both types of coarticulation, because the /b/ of *boot* is also produced with rounded lips. See Folkins and Zimmerman [1981] for similar discussion.)

Coarticulation may in certain instances be so "extreme" that the alteration in articulation produces a different phone. So far, we've seen coarticulation result in rounded consonants and nasalized vowels, changes that wouldn't alter the meaning of a word in English. /k/ produced more towards the hard palate is still perceived as the velar voiceless stop, not a /t/, which is alveolar.

Now let's consider the plural suffix on English nouns. The phoneme of the plural marker is /z/, even though it is usually written "s" in the spelling system. In a word like *dogs*, the plural suffix is pronounced as [z], the voiced fricative. For a word that ends in a voiceless sound, like *cat*, the plural is realized as [s], the voiceless counterpart to the phoneme. It is as if the –voiced feature of [t] at the end of the singular noun *cat* carries over and influences the /z/ plural phoneme marker. It is then produced as [s], as if it were sharing the voiceless feature of [t].

This extreme form of coarticulation is called *assimilation,* in which the altering of segments due to context creates a different phone. Voicing in English fricatives is distinctive and, if altered, will result in a different phone.

Coarticulation and assimilation are types of phonological processes that allow speech to be produced as rapidly as it is. Acoustically, these processes result in overlapping cues to segment identification. Nasalization in a vowel, for instance, signals the presence of a following nasal consonant. (See Ryalls, 1996, for more on acoustic consequences of context.)

SLPs should not just look at isolated phonemes; they should also consider the full word contexts and even stress and intonation patterns of utterances. Unstressed vowels, for example, tend to be pronounced as schwas (i.e., [ə]) in American English. SLPs need to know what phonological processes are present in a client's native language. What types of coarticulation can occur? When does assimilation occur? And phonological symbols such as those that designate word environments, diacritics, and so forth help to describe more exactly the phonological abilities of a client, and guide the nature of therapy to be applied.

The consonants and vowels of speech are called the *segmental elements* or *phonemes*. Speech also has a melodic component, overlaid on the segmental elements. This component is termed *suprasegmental* or *prosody* and is the subject of the next chapter.

Study Questions

1. How would you "read" the following word environments? Can you think of English words that contain these environments?

    a) #_____

    b) _____#

    c) V_____V

    d) _____N

    e) N_____

    f) #CC_____

    g) _____CC#

    h) #C_____C#

2. What would an SLP gain from differentiating between a phonetic and a phonemic level of analysis in a client's productions?

3. Look at the following words. Which ones constitute minimal pairs? What do these minimal pairs tell you about specific phonetic features in English?

    bit   Sue   nap   zoo   shoe   tap   beet

    [Hint: You may need to first transcribe these words into IPA to do the exercise.]

References

Folkins, J., & Zimmerman, G. (1981). Jaw-muscle activity during speech with the mandible fixed. *Journal of the Acoustical Society of America, 69*, 1441–1444.

Fromkin, V., & Rodman, R. (1998). *An introduction to language* (6th ed.). Fort Worth, TX: Harcourt Brace Jovanovich.

Keefe, M., & Dalton, R. (1989). An analysis of velopharyngeal timing in normal adult speakers using a microcomputer based photodetector system. *Journal of Speech and Hearing Research, 32*, 39–48.

Ladefoged, P. (1993). *A course in phonetics* (3rd ed.). Fort Worth, TX: Harcourt Brace Jovanovich.

Ryalls, J. (1996). *A basic introduction to speech perception*. San Diego, CA: Singular.

Schane, S. (1968). *French phonology and morphology*. Cambridge, MA: MIT Press.

8 Speech Prosody

Prosody has been referred to as the melody of speech (Monrad-Krohn, 1947). Although prosody has not been given the same amount of attention that segmental units of speech production have received, it is nonetheless a very important component of speech production. One way of thinking about prosody is to think of speech as a radio broadcast. In this metaphor, speech actually broadcasts two messages simultaneously. One message includes the individual phonemes or segments that allow the listener to understand the individual words being spoken. The other message is the prosody.

Hint to Students

Since *segmental* refers to the individual phoneme units of speech, *suprasegmental* is also used in addition to prosody to refer to acoustic variations over units larger than individual phonemes.

Most researchers would agree that prosody encompasses the emotional tone of a message. Speakers can convey anger, joy, or boredom through the prosodic component of speech (Ross, 1981). In fact, the linguistic content of a message can be at variance with the prosodic, as when a speaker claims that "I feel great today," in a dreary monotone.

Prosody can also supply the listener with important linguistic information (cf. Baum, 1998). This linguistic prosody can be crucial for distinguishing certain compound units that are ambiguous. For example, while *hot DOG* (with stress on the second syllable) can mean a canine who is too warm or even an exclamation of excitement on the speaker's part, *HOTdog* (stress on the first syllable) refers to the favorite snack at baseball games.

Other linguistic uses of prosody involve changes in fundamental frequency over the length of a sentence, termed intonation, as well as information about word boundaries (juncture) and the emphasis of words in a phrase or sentence.

Both types of prosody, linguistic and emotional, are produced with the same set of acoustic correlates. These acoustic components of prosody are reflected in changes in a speaker's amplitude, duration, and fundamental frequency.

This point is important: Whether a speaker is conveying linguistic information through the prosodic component of speech or is using prosody to set an emotional tone, the acoustic components at the speaker's disposal are the same: amplitude, duration, and fundamental frequency.

Hint to Students

The physiological-to-perceptual correspondence of the acoustic correlates is as follows: Amplitude is heard as volume; duration is heard as length; and fundamental frequency is heard as voice pitch. Be aware, though, that these correspondences are not necessarily linear, in that a twofold increase in f_0 may not be heard as a doubling of the speaker's pitch.

We will consider different types of linguistic prosody (sometimes called propositional prosody) and emotional (or nonpropositional) prosody in some detail below.

Linguistic Prosody

Word Stress

The placement of prosody can help determine the meaning of a word. The noun REcord, with stress on the first syllable changes to the verb reCORD when the stress shifts to the second syllable. And as seen earlier, a HOTdog is not a hotDOG. What is this phenomenon called stress?

Research into the acoustic changes that accompany the stressing of a syllable or word has shown that stress relates, as all prosodic events do, to changes in the speaker's amplitude, f_0, and duration. Moreover, it is largely the vowel in a stressed syllable that reflects these changes that are associated with prosody. In other words, if a syllable is stressed, it may well be signaled in a change in vowel length, loudness, or pitch (as perceived by the listener). Consonants show less acoustic change as a result of being in a stressed syllable. Nonetheless, many acoustic studies into the effects of stress will examine the entire syllable, not just the vowel.

Researchers have also looked at the characteristics of amplitude, f_0, and duration on syllables in general. For instance, the first syllable in a two-syllable word will tend to be higher in f_0 compared to the second syllable (Klatt, 1976). Word position (first syllable, second syllable), then, is associated with intrinsic acoustic characteristics that then interact with prosodic changes. When either a first or a final syllable is stressed, the f_0 has been found to increase, so in HOTdog, the already higher value of f_o will increase even more, resulting in a large first-to-second-syllable difference in fundamental frequency. If the second syllable is stressed, the f_o of *dog* will likely rise, but the syllable-to-syllable difference in f_o won't be as great as with *HOTdog*.

Looking at duration, final syllables in words tend to be intrinsically longer. In addition, once a syllable is stressed, it tends to lengthen. However, if the final syllable is stressed, it may not lengthen appreciably more since it started out as the longer syllable. So in *hotDOG*, the final syllable, usually lengthened because of its word position, isn't too affected by the result of stress on its duration. *HOT* in *HOTdog* would show more of a lengthening due to stress. Behrens (1988) found that many speakers signal the difference between these two types of phrases with a longer *pause* between syllables when the second syllable is stressed compared to when the first syllable is stressed.

Research has found no intrinsic characteristics of syllable position when amplitude is considered. In other words, neither first nor second syllables tend to be louder in general. Once a syllable is stressed, however, it is associated with an increase in amplitude.

Hint to Students

Particular stress patterns are associated with certain characteristics of amplitude, f_o, and duration. Particular word positions (first syllable, final syllable) are also associated with predictable acoustic traits. The two properties of stress pattern and word position interact.

Although amplitude, f_o, and duration changes are the acoustic correlates of stress, speakers don't all use the same combination of these correlates to signal such word stress. Lieberman (1960) looked at such noun/verb pairs as *REcord* and *reCORD* to see what individual speakers actually do acoustically to convey part of speech by stressing the first or the final syllable.

Lieberman found a great deal of individual variation, but some patterns emerged in the data. For example, some speakers did not use amplitude to signal stress, relying instead on f_o and duration. Others did not use f_o, employing other acoustic changes to convey the target stress pattern. However, no stressed syllable was ever lower in *both* amplitude and f_o compared to an unstressed counterpart. Further, Lieberman found f_o to be the most common acoustic change associated with stress on a syllable. In general, then, there is no one invariant pattern of acoustic changes that signals stress every time, although there are general tendencies that emerge.

Behrens (1988) also found individual differences when speakers produced such pairs as *HOTdog* and *hotDOG*. Speakers used various combinations of the three acoustic correlates of stress, and very few speakers used the same combination. In addition, she tested the listener intelligibility of using certain combinations of stress correlates and found that a particular correlate, such as f_0, used by two different speakers may not result in equally robust stress perception by listeners. In other words, one speaker may use f_0 more successfully as a stress cue, depending on the magnitude of the f_0 change.

Hint to Students

Word stress is signaled by changes in the fo, amplitude, and duration usually of the vowel segment of a syllable. Individual speakers use various combinations of these cues to stress words, although f_0 tends to be the most salient cue.

Sentence Emphasis

Prosodic changes may be employed to emphasize a word in a phrase or sentence: for example, *MARY read the book, not John*. As with word stress, emphatic stress such as this also relies on changes in the three acoustic correlates of prosody. And as with word stress, there are acoustic changes associated with emphasis that interact with the intrinsic properties of amplitude, f_0, and duration associated with certain positions in a sentence.

Words at the end of a sentence have been found to be intrinsically longer in duration than words in other sentence positions (Cooper, Eady, & Mueller, 1985). So, in *Mary read the book*, *book* (in an unemphasized reading of the sentence) would be intrinsically longer than other words. Once there is emphasis, the emphasized word, anywhere in a sentence, tends to be lengthened. Thus, in the reading *MARY read the book*, the first word would most likely lengthen because of emphasis. If the final word *book* was emphasized, it may not lengthen appreciably more since it is already intrinsically longer due to its position in the sentence.

When Cooper and colleagues investigated f_0, they found a high f_0 value associated with the first word of a sentence. If that first word were to receive an emphatic reading, the f_0 would not change measurably. Interestingly, though, words that followed were lower in f_0 than they would have been without emphasis in the sentence. So emphasis here has a more global effect on the sentence. When other words in a sentence are emphasized, they do show an increase in f_0.

Amplitude seems to be a rather weak correlate to sentence emphasis. Behrens (1988) found that amplitude was rarely used by speakers as a cue to emphasis in a sentence.

Hint to Students

As with word stress, sentence emphasis will affect words by emphasis placement and by position in the sentence. You need to consider both factors.

Sentence Intonation

Sentence intonation is defined as fluctuations in f_0 across the length of the sentence. In a sense, then, it is more global than word stress or emphasis on a single word in a sentence. When someone has a relatively flat f_0, we say that person speaks in a monotone. Speakers with "sing-songy" voices would be varying their f_0 a great deal over the course of an utterance.

There are two conflicting theories of how f_0 normally progresses across a sentence. The *declination view of intonation* (e.g., Cooper & Sorensen, 1981) proposes that f_0 gradually falls, so that each word is lower in f_0 than the previous word. This view says a plot of intonation (for a declarative sentence) would be a steady, downward sloping line.

In contrast is the *breath-group theory* (Lieberman, 1967), which considers a sentence contour not as steadily decreasing in f_0 values. Instead, the f_0 pattern is said to consist of two parts: a relatively flat preterminal f_0 pattern and a terminal portion in the last 150 to 200 milliseconds of the sentence. It is in this terminal portion that declarative sentences will differ from interrogatives. In the declarative sentence *It is raining today*, the breath-group theory predicts that the f_0 will be steady up to the last word and then fall off on the word *today*. With an interrogative sentence, the pre-terminal f_0 pattern will not differ from the declarative statement, but f_0 will remain flat or even rise on the final word *today*.

One explanation for the existence of conflicting theories of intonation may be the widely different ways researchers measure f_0 changes, and the fact that some studies analyze read speech while others look at spontaneous utterances; they may not be comparable (see Behrens, 1989).

Hint to Students

The two views of sentence intonation predict either a steadily falling f_0 throughout the sentence (declination view) or a relatively stable f_0 with steep f_0 fall-off at the end of the sentence (breath-group theory).

Emotional Prosody

Changes in f_0, duration, and amplitude are used to signal linguistic information: parts of speech, different phrases, emphasis, and sentence types. But these same three acoustic parameters can be manipulated to signal affect—convey an emotional message in an utterance.

Williams and Stevens (1972) looked at the acoustic changes that accompany sentences that sound sad, joyful, and so on. They used trained actors, but other researchers have used spontaneous speech that was full of emotion, even including the radio broadcast of the Hindenburg explosion, where the announcer was clearly very distraught.

As with individual differences in conveying linguistic prosody, emotional prosody can't be absolutely categorized by emotion and acoustic trait, such as "to sound angry, raise your amplitude by 10 dB and f_o by 50 Hz." (One of us remembers a fourth grade teacher who showed her displeasure with the class by speaking more quietly and lowering the pitch of her voice.)

Most research on emotional prosody has actually been conducted on individuals who have suffered damage to the right cerebral hemisphere. Clinical impressions find right hemisphere damaged (RHD) speakers speaking in a monotone, unable to express emotion. Many researchers have found a similar problem among RHD populations in trying to convey the emotional content of speech (cf. Bloom, Borod, Obler, & Gerstwan, 1992) as well as identifying the emotions being conveyed in an utterance (Borod, Andelman, Obler, Tweedy, & Welkowitz, 1992).

Neurological Representation of Prosody and Dysprosody

Because emotional and linguistic prosody are conveyed by the same set of acoustic correlates, researchers have proposed that prosody of any kind must be located in the same part of the brain. And because of reported deficits in conveying prosody, at least the emotional kind, in RHD speakers, the right hemisphere has been hypothesized to be the neurological site of prosody in general (Heilman, Bowers, Speedie, & Coslett, 1984; Ross, 1981).

Another hypothesis, the *functional load hypothesis*, posits a right-hemisphere site for emotional prosody and a left-hemisphere site for linguistic prosody (Behrens, 1985; Van Lancker, 1980). The linguistic function of the prosody will thus determine which hemisphere is engaged in producing or perceiving the changes in f_o, amplitude, and duration.

Finally, recent studies have proposed that each hemisphere processes a different acoustic correlate, at least for linguistic prosody. The left hemisphere seems more involved in the processing of temporal aspects of prosody, such as duration cues, while the right hemisphere is better suited to processing f_o changes (Van Lancker & Sidtis, 1992; cf. Baum, 1998). Ryalls (1982) challenges this view, however, because he found certain *left*-hemisphere damaged individuals with a fluency disorder to have monotonous intonation (f_o contours).

The research continues. It may well be that the two hemispheres of the brain are not working separately, but instead are integrating information, both linguistic and affective. In chapter 13, we return to the neurological representation of speech. First, we will examine various ways that the acoustic correlates of speech in general are measured.

Study Questions

1. What are the acoustic/physical correlates of prosody and their perceptual/psychological associates?

2. Explain the difference between linguistic and emotional prosody.

3. What is the current view on the neurological representation of prosody? Discuss both the right and left hemispheres.

4. Discuss the viewpoint of the breath-group theory of intonation. How does it differ from the declination view?

References

Baum, S. (1998). The role of fundamental frequency and duration in the perception of linguistic stress by individuals with brain damage. *Journal of Speech, Language, and Hearing Research, 41,* 31–40.

Behrens, S. (1985). The perception of stress and lateralization of prosody. *Brain and Language, 26,* 332–348.

Behrens, S. (1988). The role of the right hemisphere in the production of linguistic stress. *Brain and Language, 33,* 104–127.

Behrens, S. (1989). Characterizing sentence intonation in a right hemisphere damaged population. *Brain and Language, 37,* 181–200.

Bloom, R., Borod, J., Obler, L., & Gerstman, L. (1992). Impact of emotional content on discourse production in patients with unilateral brain damage. *Brain and Language, 42,* 153–164.

Borod, J., Andelman, F., Obler, L., Tweedy, J., & Welkowitz, J. 1992. Right hemisphere specialization for the identification of emotional words and sentences: Evidence from stroke patients. *Neuropsychologia, 30,* 827–844.

Cooper, W., Eady, S., & Mueller, P. (1985). Acoustic aspects of contrastive stress in question-answer contexts. *Journal of the Acoustical Society of America, 77,* 2124–2156.

Cooper, W., & Sorensen, J. (1981). *Fundamental frequency in sentence production.* New York: Springer Verlag.

Heilman, K., Bowers, D., Speedie, L., & Coslett, H. (1984). Comprehension of affective and non-affective prosody. *Neurology, 34,* 917–920.

Klatt, D. (1976). Linguistic uses of duration in English: Acoustic and perceptual evidence. *Journal of the Acoustical Society of America, 59,* 1208–1221.

Lieberman, P. (1960). Some acoustic correlates of word stress in American English. *Journal of the Acoustical Society of America, 32,* 451–454.

Lieberman, P. (1967). *Intonation, perception and language.* Cambridge, MA: MIT Press.

Monrad-Krohn, G. (1947). Dysprosody or altered "melody of language." *Brain, 70,* 405–415.

Ross, E. (1981). The aprosodias: Functional-anatomical organization of the affective components of language in the right hemisphere. *Archives of Neurology, 38,* 561–569.

Ryalls, J. (1982). Intonation in Broca's aphasia. *Neuropsychologia, 20,* 355–360.

Van Lancker, D. (1980). Cerebral lateralization of pitch cues in the linguistic signal. *International Journal of Human Communication, 13,* 227–277.

Van Lancker, D., & Sidtis, J. (1992). The identification of affective-prosodic stimuli by left- and right-hemisphere-damaged subjects: All errors are not created equal. *Journal of Speech and Hearing Research, 35,* 963–970.

Williams, C., & Stevens, K. 1972. Emotions and speech: Some acoustic correlates. *Journal of the Acoustical Society of America, 52,* 1238–1250.

CHAPTER

9

Acoustic Measures of Speech

A rather astonishing array of acoustic measures has been applied to speech. Acoustic measures of speech are much more common than physiological measures because they are noninvasive. That is, they are not uncomfortable because they do not "invade" or restrain the human body in the way that electrodes being inserted into muscle fibers or a mask being held against the face would. In fact, usually they are performed on previously recorded speech, so any analysis is typically performed long after the speaker has left the speech laboratory. Some acoustic studies have included measures from speech that was recorded over forty years ago!

While we will not consider all of the possible acoustic measures of speech, we will discuss those of major importance to speech language pathology and audiology. By and large, acoustic measures of speech can conveniently be divided into two types: *temporal* measures and *frequency* measures. There are also measures of *intensity*, which listeners perceive as loudness. But in most measures of speech, we are interested in the intensity at particular frequencies of speech, so intensity will not be discussed further here.

Temporal Measures

The primary temporal measure of speech is *duration*. The duration of speech can be measured as broadly as a total sentence duration, or as minutely as the duration of a single period of phonation. However, word-, syllable-, and phoneme-sized duration measures are most common and relevant to speech. When the number of syllables or words is measured in reference to some unit of time (typically seconds or minutes), speech rate, another duration measure, can be derived. It is perhaps somewhat more accurate to measure speech rate in syllables per second than words per minute, since a word can easily vary from one to five or more syllables in length.

Although crude measures of speech rate can be derived from a simple stopwatch, a stopwatch is not considered accurate enough for research purposes.

Hint to Students

Duration is an acoustic correlate, usually measured in milliseconds, and perceived as length.

Stopwatch measures may be useful in collecting preliminary clinical data such as the rate at which a speaker can alternate simple syllables such as /pa/, /ta/, /ka/ (known as the *diadochokinetic rate*). These data can then be compared to published averages and ranges for normal speakers such as Kent (1994). However, while one can become fairly skilled at stopping and starting a stopwatch, it still takes a small amount of time for the brain to receive a speech signal and then send a command to the finger to depress the stopwatch. Measures of speech rate using a stopwatch are likely to include this "reaction time."

Voice onset time (VOT) is another important duration measure. It is related to the difference between voiced and voiceless stop consonants. That is, VOT relates to the difference between voiced stop consonants such as /b/, /d/, and /g/ and their voiceless counterparts /p/, /t/, and /k/. VOT assesses the time between two articulatory events: the opening of the vocal tract after complete obstruction associated with the production of stop consonants and the onset of vocal fold vibration. Of course, the VOT is longer for a voiceless stop consonant than it is for a voiced stop consonant. (See Figures 5.2, 5.3, and 5.4 in chapter 5 where VOT is also discussed.) This increased delay in vocal fold vibration after stop release is perceived by listeners as voicelessness. The VOT value would be positive. The vocal folds can also begin vibration <u>before</u> the release of the consonant, in which case the VOT is negative. Negative VOT is also known as *prevoicing*. Although prevoicing for voiced stop consonants is not considered to be typical of American English, the normal speaker of American English does occasionally produce some voiced stops with negative VOT values. In fact, some of our own research has shown more negative VOT productions in the speech of American speakers of English than previous studies have suggested (Ryalls, Zipprer, & Bauldauff, 1997).

VOT is a popular measure that has been investigated in a wide variety of speech disorders. Some of these disorders include hearing impairment (e.g., Monsen, 1976; Ryalls & Larouche, 1992), adult aphasia (e.g., Blumstein, Cooper, Goodglass, Statlender, & Gottlieb, 1980), and dysarthria (e.g., Morris, 1989). The normal acquisition of the voicing distinction in children has also been investigated

Hint to Students

VOT is a measurement of time that elapses between stop release and vocal fold vibration. A long positive VOT value is associated with voiceless stops; a short positive 0 or negative VOT value is associated with voiced stops.

(e.g., Kewley-Port & Preston, 1974). Behrens, Anderson, and Sidtis (1987) found abnormal VOT values for stop consonants in the production of individuals with a cerebellar disorder. Specifically, patients failed to make clear distinctions between voiced and voiceless stops. An impairment in coordination was implicated.

The process of normal aging also seems to affect VOT production (Ryalls, Cliche, Fortier-Blanc, Coulombe, & Prudhommeaux, 1997; Sweeting & Baken, 1981). Some studies have found that VOT is affected by gender, ethnic background, and native language of the speaker (Ryalls, Zipprer, & Baldauff, 1997; Thornburgh & Ryalls, 1998). Hoit, Solomon, and Hixon (1993) have also found a significant correlation between VOT and lung volume, suggesting that the production of VOT is constrained by physiology as well as by the linguistic purpose of voicing contrasts.

But all of these studies are somewhat limited in scope and preliminary in nature. These VOT studies of various speech disorders need to be replicated with larger groups of speakers. More work on the normal production of voice onset time would also provide a better basis for comparison with various speech disorders. With computer-based speech analysis systems becoming ever more powerful, perhaps even fully automatized VOT measures are not too far off in the future. Such automatized VOT measures may also eventually contribute to convenient screening procedures for clients at-risk for certain speech disorders.

Frequency Measures

The most basic frequency measure for speech is the fundamental frequency (i.e., the rate of vocal fold vibration). Listeners hear the fundamental frequency as the pitch of a speaker's voice, as was discussed in chapter 4 on phonation. We all know that male voices are typically much lower sounding than female voices. Listeners hear the up and down variation of the fundamental frequency as a speaker's intonation, which was discussed in chapter 8 on prosody.

Hint to Students

Frequency is a physical acoustic correlate, usually measured in Hertz, that is perceived as pitch.

The frequency measures that pertain most directly to the differences between the various speech sounds are the first and second formant frequencies (e.g., F_1, F_2). Since recognizable speech can be synthesized with only two formants, the first and second formant frequencies are the most important frequency differences relevant to speech.

There are other frequency measures related to formant frequency values. For example, the frequency range and timing of formant frequency transitions are also important acoustic measures for speech. Figure 6.3 in chapter 6 gave a schematic of a formant, illustrating the difference between the steady-state portion and the transition portion. In a general sense, the steady-state portion of a formant relates more to the vowel portion of a syllable, while the formant transition relates more to the consonant portion.

Second frequency (F_2) transitions have been especially implicated in providing listeners with information on place of articulation, distinguishing between [b] and [d], for example. However, F_2 transitions alone cannot provide sufficient acoustic information for uniquely specifying place of articulation for a particular consonant in various vowel contexts. In other words, there is no one invariant frequency transition property associated with any particular consonant combined in syllables with all vowels. This lack of explanatory power is sometimes referred to as the problem of acoustic invariance. But we would have to consider the process of speech perception in much more detail in order to discuss this issue. (See Ryalls, 1996, for a discussion of acoustic invariance.)

Equipment to Measure Frequency and Temporal Characteristics

Spectrographs and Spectrograms

One piece of equipment that allows researchers to measure the frequency and temporal characteristics of speech is the sound spectrograph. The *spectrograph* is a machine that produces a "picture" of speech called a *spectrogram*. A spectrogram depicts the frequency changes in speech over time. Amplitude, although not an axis in traditional spectrograms, is indicated by the darkness of the image. Figure 9.1 is a photograph of a Kay Digital spectrograph, and Figure 9.2 is an example of a spectrographic printout.

Hint to Students

Spectrograph or sonagraph is the name of the machine that produces a spectrogram or a sonagram. You can remember this if you think that a telegram is the thing that people read, while the telegraph is the machine that it is sent on.

Spectrograms analyze speech at particular bandwidths depending on the filter setting that is used. Narrow filters allow the user to observe the harmonics in the narrowband spectrogram that results. With the wide filter setting, wideband spectrograms are produced that tend not to capture individual harmonics. Wideband spectrograms are used more than narrowband spectrograms because they

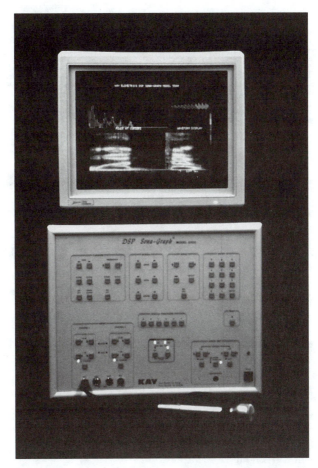

FIGURE 9.1   Photograph of a Kay Elemetrics Digital Sonagraph. (Reprinted with permission from Kay Elemetrics Corporation.)

are somewhat more sensitive to timing changes and they allow more accurate measures of formant frequencies. Figure 9.2 is a printout of the computer screen from a Kay Elemetrics CSL spectrographic image. In the topmost portion is the raw waveform of the sentence "We were away a year ago." Below it is a wideband spectrogram of the sentence, while the lowest portion is the narrowband spectrogram of the same sentence.

Computer-Based Systems

Although the sound spectrograph was formerly the only method available for measuring formant frequencies of speech, computer-based formant frequency extraction is becoming more and more popular because it offers several distinct advantages. The foremost advantage is that the computer also often performs the

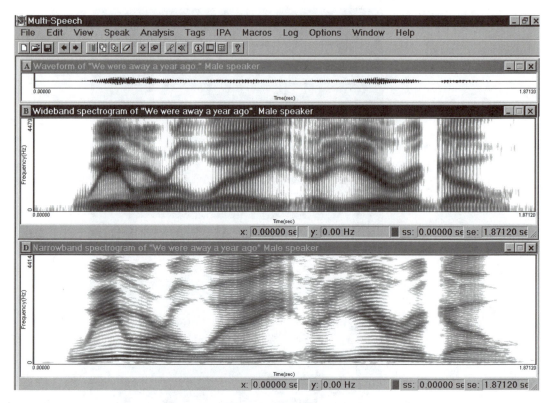

FIGURE 9.2   Spectrograms of the sentence "We were away a year ago" spoken by an adult male speaker. The waveform appears in the upper portion of the computer printout. Below it is a wideband spectrogram, and a narrowband spectrogram appears below it. (Reprinted with permission from Kay Elemetrics Corporation.)

extrapolation of formant values. Formerly, actual formant frequency values had to be extrapolated by hand from a sound spectrogram. In fact, obtaining the spectrogram is only the first step in obtaining formant frequency measures by spectrograph (as anyone who has performed a large number of these measures by the spectrograph knows all too well!). However, the popularity of computers also seems to have resulted in a reduction in the use of spectrograms for deriving formant frequency values, even when the spectrogram is produced by a computer.

Most contemporary computer systems employ linear predictive coding (or LPC) as the mathematical algorithm for deriving the frequency values of formants (Atal & Hanauer, 1971). While a Fourier analysis provides a rough indication of formant frequencies of speech as discussed in chapter 6, an LPC analysis is required to derive the actual formant frequency values. (Figure 6.2 was an example of a LPC spectrum for a /i/ vowel produced by a normal adult speaker, and Table 6.1 listed some average formant values for three different vowels.)

While the most widely used computer speech analysis system in the laboratories of speech-language pathology departments these days is undoubtedly the Kay Elemetrics Computer Speech System (CSL), Cspeech (Milenkovic, 1989) and the Barus Laboratory Interactive Speech System (BLISS) (Mertus, 1989) have also been employed in a large number of published research articles. Reviews of several different PC-based speech analysis systems can be found in Read, Budner, and Kent (1990) and Ryalls and Baum (1990). The use of computers will be discussed in further detail in chapter 17.

Although there are many other frequency measures available (such as a weighting of the LPC spectrum, called the *centroid*, and bark measures), formant frequency measures will always remain the foremost frequency measures for speech because they are the primary acoustic properties of speech.

Jitter and Shimmer

There are two other important measures related to the fundamental frequency—*jitter* and *shimmer*. These measures are discussed here and not with the fundamental frequency because they are not as popular measures of speech as are VOT and formant frequency measures. Typically, they are used more often in studies of voice disorders.

Jitter is a measure of the way that the vibration of the vocal folds varies from one cycle of vibration to the next. Since jitter assesses period-to-period duration variation, it is actually a temporal measure. Shimmer is a measure of the way that the amplitude varies from one period of the fundamental frequency to the next. Thus it is an amplitude measure. See Figures 9.3 and 9.4 for an illustration of the difference between jitter and shimmer.

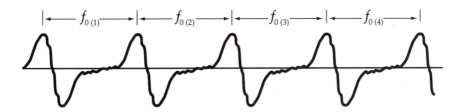

FIGURE 9.3 Schematic of a speech waveform with the periods marked. Jitter refers to the average variation in the fundamental frequency compared from one period to the next. Jitter is also known as "frequency perturbation."

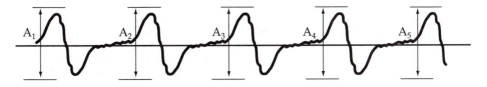

FIGURE 9.4 Schematic of a speech waveform with the periods marked. Shimmer refers to the average variation in the amplitude compared from one period to the next. Shimmer is also known as "amplitude perturbation."

Assessing Voice Disorders

Jitter, shimmer, and other measures have been shown to relate to voicing. The Computer Speech Lab (CSL) from Kay Elemetrics offers a variety of such voice measures in its Multi-Dimensional Voice Profile (MDVP) program. "Voicing" or "phonation" refers to the vibration pattern of the vocal folds. Phonation measures may be useful in assessing various voice disorders. These measures often reflect when the voice is not working in an optimal manner due to problems such as vocal nodules, which prevent a typical complete closing of the vocal folds.

An inappropriate sounding voice (i.e., fundamental frequency too low or too high) or an abnormally raspy, hoarse, or breathy voice can be the first indications of a voicing problem. A common first step in assessing a voice disorder is to obtain an average fundamental frequency measure for a voice client, and then to compare this value to published values such as Colton and Casper (1996). Behrman and Orlikoff (1997) outline a method of using measures to refine a treatment plan for voice disorders. However, most students learn a lot more information on vocal fold vibration in an entire course devoted to Voice. Further discussion of voice measures is beyond the scope of this introductory text.

In the next chapter, we examine physiological measures of speech production. These measures are different from acoustic measures in that they are derived directly from the speaker and not from the acoustic speech output. It is important to bear in mind that the sound that is measured in acoustic measures is the result of the movements of speech structures. In the next chapter, we will consider direct measures of the movement of speech structures.

Study Questions

1. What type of duration measures are available to speech scientists?

2. Name some common frequency measures used in speech analysis.

3. Define VOT and explain why it is an important measure for SLPs.

4. What is the significance of the F_1 and F_2 values of vowels? Why are these measures relevant to speech therapy?

References

Atal, B., & Hanauer, S. (1971). Speech analysis and synthesis by linear prediction of the speech wave. *Journal of the Acoustical Society of America, 50,* 637–655.

Behrens, S., Anderson, N., & Sidtis, J. (1987). The control of voice onset time and vowel duration after paraneoplastic cerebellar degeneration. *Journal of the Acoustical Society of America, 82,* S18.

Behrman, A., & Orlikoff, R. (1997). Instrumentation in voice assessment and treatment: What's the use? *American Journal of Speech-Language Pathology, 6,* 9–16.

Blumstein, S., Cooper, W., Goodglass, H., Statlender, S. & Gottlieb, J. (1980). Production deficits in aphasia: A voice-onset time analysis. *Brain and Language, 9*, 153–170.

Colton, R., & Casper, J. (1996). *Understanding voice problems: A physiological perspective for diagnosis and treatment* (2nd ed.). Baltimore, MD: Williams & Wilkins.

Hoit, J., Solomon, P., & Hixon, T. (1993). Effect of lung volume on voice onset time (VOT). *Journal of Speech and Hearing Research, 36*, 516–521.

Kent, R. (1994). *Reference manual for communicative sciences and disorders*. Austin, TX: Pro-Ed.

Kewley-Port, D., & Preston, M. 1974. Early apical stop production: A voice-onset time analysis. *Journal of Phonetics, 2*, 195–210.

Mertus, J. (1989). *BLISS User Manual*. Providence, RI: Brown University.

Milenkovic, P. (1989). *Cspeech: Computer software waveform acquisition, editing and analysis*. Madison, WI: University of Wisconsin.

Monsen, R. (1976). The production of English stop consonants in the speech of deaf children. *Journal of Phonetics, 4*, 29–42.

Morris, R. (1989). VOT and dysarthria: A descriptive study. *Journal of Communication Disorders, 22*, 23–33.

Read, C., Budner, E., & Kent, R. 1990. Speech analysis systems: A survey. *Journal of Speech and Hearing Research, 33(2)*, 363–374.

Ryalls, J. (1996). *A basic introduction to speech perception*. San Diego, CA: Singular.

Ryalls, J., & Baum, S. (1990). Review of three software systems for speech analysis: Cspeech, BLISS and CSRE. *Journal of Speech-Language Pathology and Audiology, 14(3)*, 49–52.

Ryalls, J., Cliche, A., Fortier-Blanc, J., Coulombe, I., & Prudhommeaux, A. (1997). Voice-onset time in younger and older French-speaking Canadians. *Clinical Linguistics and Phonetics, 11(3)*, 205–212.

Ryalls, J., & Larouche, A. (1992). Acoustic integrity of speech production in children with moderate and severe hearing impairment. *Journal of Speech and Hearing Research, 35*, 88–95.

Ryalls, J., Zipprer, A., & Baldauff, A. (1997). A preliminary investigation of the effects of gender and race on voice onset time. *Journal of Speech, Language, and Hearing Research, 40*, 642–645.

Sweeting, P., & Baken, R. (1982). Voice onset time in a normal-aged population. *Journal of Speech and Hearing Research, 25*, 129–134.

Thornburgh, D., & Ryalls, J. (1998). Voice onset time in Spanish-English bilinguals: Early versus late learners of English. *Journal of Communication Disorders, 31*, 215–229.

CHAPTER

10 Physiological Measures of Speech

We turn now to a discussion of the means of speech production, specifically the way that the physiology involved in speaking is measured. This discussion includes measurements of the muscle tension and movement involved in articulation, the electrical activity in these muscles, and related changes in human anatomy. There are also air flow and air pressure measures pertaining to different aspects of speech production.

There is somewhat less research employing physiological measures than there is using acoustic measures. Physiological measures are, quite simply, more difficult to obtain. Such research typically requires the physical presence of the speaker, as well as relatively expensive and oftentimes delicate equipment. Physiological measures also require personnel with more specialized training than is the case with most common acoustic measures of speech. Finally, physiological measures can involve the insertion of electrode wires directly into speakers' muscles and may thus require the presence of medical personnel.

Despite the greater difficulty in acquiring physiological measures, they are sometimes preferred because they relate to speech production in a much more direct manner. Very few acoustic measures of speech relate directly to its physical production—there is typically a rather complex relationship between articulation and its effect in the resulting acoustic signal. We will consider measures of respiration, articulation, and laryngeal activity.

Respiration

Respiration can be assessed through strain belts, which are placed on the chest to measure chest wall displacement. Electronic transducers can also be placed on the chest to measure chest wall displacement. The pneumotachograph is a mask placed over the nose and face that is outfitted with sensors connected to a computer system to measure air flow during various speech tasks. Sapienza and Dutka (1996) have used the pneumotachograph to investigate changes in glottal airflow characteristics in female speakers across various age groups.

Articulation

The full array of physiological measures in articulation cannot be considered in an introductory text. However, some of the most important physiological measures of speech will be considered below. Two of the most important are two different types of muscle tension recordings. Muscle tension is measured in such recordings because muscle tension does not always result in movement. It is measured by means of electromyographic recordings. These recordings are of two different forms—one type is recorded from the skin surface, the other type is recorded from within the muscle.

Hint to Students

Electromyographic (EMG) recordings are used to measure electrical (electro) activity associated with muscle (myo) tension, and they take the form of a continuous line (graph).

Electromyography is abbreviated as EMG. In *surface EMG*, sensing electrodes are affixed to the surface of the skin. These electrodes are used to record the activity of the muscles below where they are placed. They are simply taped or temporarily "glued" to the surface of the skin with a light removable adhesive. In the other type of EMG, known as *intramuscular EMG*, small thin wires are inserted directly into the muscle fiber. This can be somewhat uncomfortable since they must be inserted with a hypodermic needle, and this procedure may require the presence of a licensed physician when the structures of speech are involved. This type of myography is also known as *hooked wire EMG*, because the tiny wires that are inserted into the muscle have a small hook or bend in the wire so that they stay secured in the muscle for the duration of the recording session. A slight tug on the wires at the end of the recording session straightens the wires and pulls them loose from the muscles (Gay & Harris, 1971).

There are advantages and disadvantages to each of these two procedures. Surface EMG is noninvasive. The only uncomfortable part of this procedure can be the mild abrasion of the skin surface to remove oil and dead skin cells in order to reduce the electrical impedance and optimize the EMG recording. This exfoliation may also serve to improve the adhesion of the electrodes. The reduced invasiveness of surface EMG recordings tends to make for much more willing volunteers than the direct insertion method. Oftentimes in the past, researchers had to perform intramuscular EMG recordings upon themselves or their research colleagues, since willing participants were sometimes difficult to recruit.

However, because glued or taped recording electrodes only sit on the surface of skin, they are less accurate in isolating the activity of a single muscle. It is often impossible to be sure that activity from a single muscle is indeed being recorded. It should be pointed out, however, that there has been considerable improvement in the sensitivity of surface electrodes so that surface EMG recordings have become quite sensitive. Since a single wire may be inserted into a particular muscle, it is much more likely with the *hooked wire method* that the activity of a single muscle fiber is being measured.

EMG recordings can be performed on almost any of the myriad of muscles involved in the complex muscular activity of speech, provided that a means of access can be found. For example, it is practically impossible to attach surface electrodes to the rapidly moving and highly malleable tongue—at least in a manner that does not greatly limit mobility and consequently interfere with normal speech production.

Hint to Students

The two types of EMG recordings are (1) surface EMG, using electrodes glued, or taped, over muscles; and (2) intramuscular or hooked wire EMG, involving wires inserted into muscles.

A method for viewing tongue contact with the palate is that of *electropalatography* (EPG). In this method a subject is fitted with an acrylic mold of the palate, called a pseudo-palate, in which tiny sensing electrodes have been placed. A computer system can then be used to record the contact of the tongue with various positions on the hard and soft palate.

Movement of the articulators can be captured and observed using several other techniques. Microbeam X-rays employ an X-ray beam and computer system to isolate and track radio-sensitive markers attached to various articulators. While subjects produce various speech sounds, articulation can be observed and recorded. It is then possible to review speech movements in detail in several dimensions.

In ultrasound measures, high-frequency sound waves are generated by a transducer placed adjacent to an articulatory area. As with sonar used by submarines and air-traffic control systems, sound waves echo back when they make contact with objects. These echoed signals can then be used to convey a view of cavities and structures in the vocal tract, and how they change during speech production. These days, a similar system is used to view the developing fetus in a pregnant mother. Such systems are sensitive enough to determine the gender of the future child and reveal problems in development of the essential organs. An ultrasound method that allows three-dimensional views has also recently been developed.

A relatively new method of exploring articulation that is currently gaining popularity is that of *electromagnetic articulography* (EMA). In this method small sensing coils are temporarily fixed to a speaker's articulators (such as the tongue and lips), which can then be recorded and tracked by computer. The computer system can then be used to reconstruct the speaker's articulatory movements. This system allows researchers to view articulation, which previously could not be seen because it occurred inside the mouth and vocal tract, in three dimensions. Carstens Medizinelektronik Company in Germany has commercialized such a system. A photograph of such a system, supplied by Carstens, is shown in Figure 10.1. Additional information about the Articulograph can be obtained by contacting the Carstens' website at http://www.articulograph.de, and there is a lot of useful information about using the system and how it works at http://www. humnet.ucla.edu/humnet/linguistics/facilities/physiology/ema.html (a website maintained by the Phonetics Lab of the Department of Linguistics at the University of California at Los Angeles [UCLA]).

Quite recently, another new technique for observing ongoing speech production has been developed. This technique is called *functional or dynamic magnetic resonance imaging* (fMRI). In MRI imaging, a very strong magnet temporarily displaces the orientation of subatomic particles in the molecules of the body. This temporary displacement can be picked up by sensitive detectors and used by a

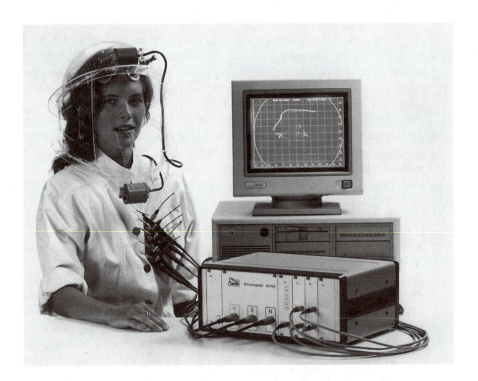

FIGURE 10.1   Photograph of a speaker outfitted with a Carstens articulograph. The articulography method is also known as electromagnetic articulography or EMA. (Reprinted by permission from Carstens Medizinelektronik GmbH.)

computer to construct an image of the structures under observation. Early MRI systems were used to derive detailed static images of the body and brain that are used to diagnose various disorders. fMRI allows for a picture of rapidly moving articulators. More discussion of MRI and the brain, as well as an example of a MRI image will be found in chapter 13. MRI images are often preferred over X-rays since they do not involve exposing the body to radiation and they may be much clearer than previous imaging systems. Strong electromagnetic fields are currently not known to have detrimental effects on the body.

A complete list of physiological measures of speech production should not overlook the relatively low-cost two-dimensional strain gauges that are still popular for recording movements of the upper lip, lower lip, and jaw during speech. One such system has been used to investigate various motor speech impairments (Barlow & Abbs, 1983). Technology is advancing rapidly in this area indeed, and it is difficult to keep pace with developments in physiological recording and imaging techniques. Table 10.1 summarizes physiological measures of speech articulators. There is more detailed current information on physiological measures of speech in Kent (1997). We now turn to physiological measures of laryngeal activity.

TABLE 10.1   Physiological Measures of Articulators in Speech Production

Type	What Is Measured
Surface EMG	Activity of muscle below electrode
Intramuscular EMG	Activity of muscle in which wire is inserted
EPG	Contact of tongue with hard and soft palate
Microbeam X-rays	Markers on articulators track movement
Ultrasound	Sound waves sensitive to structure density
Articulograph (EMA)	Sensing coils on articulators are tracked by computer in three dimensions
fMRI	Magnetic field displaces molecules and allows detailed dynamic images
Strain gauge	Noninvasive recording of lip and jaw displacement

Laryngeal Activity

One type of physiological recording for the vocal folds is known as *electroglottography*, or EGG, and is specific to the muscles of the larynx. Small transducers are attached on either side of the throat above the larynx. When correctly positioned, these transducers register changes in electrical impedance that are thought to be directly correlated with the systematic increases and decreases in vocal fold contact areas that result from phonation. The EGG method of measuring the fundamental frequency (or rate of vocal fold vibration) may, under some conditions, be more accurate than an acoustic method. This is because the acoustic signal also contains the effects of the supralaryngeal vocal tract on the fundamental frequency. In some cases, the manner in which the vocal tract filters or shapes the acoustic signal can obscure the fundamental frequency (e.g., when there is not a large difference between the fundamental frequency and the first resonance or first formant frequency, F_1). However, it is not always possible to obtain a strong and accurate EGG signal in all subjects.

There are other physiological measures of laryngeal activity that do not measure electrical activity. Instead, they involve motion pictures or video images, X-rays, and photographs. One can, for example, observe vocal fold activity by means of a small mirror positioned at the back of the throat above the vocal folds. This technique, using a laryngeal mirror, was first developed by Manuel Garcia in 1854 (Kent, 1997). The activity of the vocal folds can also be observed through an endoscopic evaluation of the larynx. An endoscope is a small camera that conducts an image to a lens where it can be observed directly. An image may also be conducted through a fiberoptic cable to a video recorder where it can then be recorded. The endoscope itself can either be rigid or flexible. A rigid endoscope must be inserted through the open mouth and positioned almost directly over the vocal folds so that they can be viewed and their activity recorded. Since it is inserted in the mouth, it interferes with ongoing speech production—especially with the production of consonants that require a closing gesture of the vocal tract. A flexible endoscope may be used to obtain an unobstructed view of speech production. However, it must be inserted through one of the nares (nostrils) and exit through the velopharyngeal port. This type of endoscope has a flexible end that can be controlled by a small dial to move in a particular direction to help guide insertion. Some people find this an uncomfortable procedure, and so a topical anesthetic is typically applied before attempting insertion of a flexible endoscope. The advantage of the flexible endoscope is that since the mouth can be closed, it allows a view of the vocal folds in connected speech. Since the subject cannot close the mouth with the rigid endoscope in place, vocal fold vibration can only be observed during the production of a sustained vowel and not during unimpeded connected speech.

Another method of observing vocal fold vibration, *cinematography*, uses high-speed camera work to film the abduction and adduction of the folds. If filmed with a flashing strobe light, vocal fold vibration appears to be moving in slow motion. This photographic technique is called *stroboscopy*. The strobe method can also be combined with slower viewing of the video recordings to further slow down the rapid vibration of the vocal folds. Since the vocal folds vibrate so rapidly, usually more than 100 times a second, they appear to be blurred to the human eye, and a method for slowing down this vibration is required to observe the opening and closing pattern in more detail. See Table 10.2 for a summary of physiological measures of vocal fold activity.

TABLE 10.2 **Physiological Measures of Vocal Fold Activity**

Type	Method of Observation
EGG	Transducers on throat record electrical activity
Endoscope	Small camera in VT records vocal fold vibration
Cinematography	High-speed moving pictures of vocal fold vibration
Stroboscopy	Moving pictures of vocal fold vibration with strobe light to appear to slow down movement

In the next chapter, we will be considering hearing, which is another important component of human communication. Our physiological investigation will continue there with a discussion of the anatomy of the human ear and auditory system.

Study Questions

1. What are the advantages and disadvantages to physiological measures of speech compared to acoustic measures?

2. Describe two types of physiological measures of muscle activity during speech.

3. Describe two types of measures of vocal fold vibration.

4. Describe two types of measures of articulation in speech.

References

Barlow, S., & Abbs, J. (1983). Force transducers for the evaluation of the labial, lingual, and mandibular motor impairments. *Journal of Speech and Hearing Research, 16,* 248–256.

Gay, T., & Harris, K. (1971). Some recent developments in the use of electromyography in speech research. *Journal of Speech and Hearing Research, 14,* 241–246.

Kent, R. (1997). *The speech sciences.* San Diego, CA: Singular.

Sapienza, C., & Dutka, J. (1996). Glottal airflow characteristics of women's voice production along an aging continuum. *Journal of Speech and Hearing Research, 39,* 322–328.

CHAPTER

11 Hearing

As human listeners it is essential that we have intact hearing in order to understand speech. But we tend to take hearing for granted, and it may only be when we begin to lose our hearing that we understand the serious role it plays in both the reception and production of speech. While we are all aware that we could not perceive spoken language without hearing, we might be less mindful of the serious compromise to the production of speech that can be the result of a serious hearing impairment.

Although the present text has placed a greater emphasis on the speech production side of the speaker-listener dyad, speech-language pathologists need to be aware of the role that hearing plays in speech. Therefore, we will review the hearing process. Most students of speech-language pathology, and certainly audiology students, will receive much more detailed instruction on the hearing process from courses in audiology and hearing science.

Hearing is the means by which the sound waves in the air are captured by the listener's sensory system. Ultimately, hearing is the process by which physical perturbations of air particles are transformed into neural impulses. It is useful to consider two separate levels of this process. The first level of the hearing process pertains to the ear. The second level of this process, where auditory signals are matched with linguistic representations, pertains to the brain. In the present text, we refer to the first level as *hearing* and to the second level as *perception*. Chapter 12 discusses speech perception.

Structure of the Ear and the Nature of Hearing

The outermost part of the ear is called the *pinna*. This is where the earlobe is found. The pinna acts to direct sound into the auditory canal. Have you ever noticed how people sometimes use their hand to funnel sounds into the ear to hear better, or as a gesture to signal the speaker to speak more loudly? The pinna acts as a kind of funnel for sound. The pinna and the *external auditory canal* make up the outer ear. In the boundary between the outer and the middle ear, the pressure displacements of the sound waves are transformed into displacements of the *tympanic membrane,* more commonly known as the *eardrum.* These physical displacements are conveyed and amplified by the three tiny bones of the middle ear: the *malleus* (hammer), the *incus* (anvil), and the *stapes* (stirrup).

These three bones are the tiniest bones of the human body. They are sometimes referred to as *ossicles,* derived from Latin for little bones, due to their small size. These bones act somewhat like a lever and not only convey the physical displacements of the eardrum, but also serve to magnify them to a considerable degree. The last bone of the ossicular chain, the stapes, attaches directly to the *cochlea.* Also in the middle ear is the *eustachian tube,* which leads to the *nasalpharyngeal cavity* and aids in maintaining relative air pressure on both sides of the tympanic membrane.

The cochlea, part of the inner ear, is shaped like a spiraling nautilus shell. It is filled with a fluid that influences hearing and as well as balance. Along the floor of the cochlea is the *basilar membrane.* If unwound and stretched out straight, the basilar membrane can be seen to be wider at one end. Somewhat counterintuitively, this wider end is more pliable than the more narrow end. Because of this difference in pliability, different sound frequencies cause the basilar membrane to react at different points along its length. The basilar membrane reacts to lower frequencies at the wider end, while higher frequencies stimulate the more narrow end. Figure 11.1 depicts the cochlea with its tonotopic arrangement. The electrical signals sent to the brain, which are already arranged by frequency by the basilar membrane, also preserve some degree of this organization by frequency when they are delivered to the *auditory cortex.*

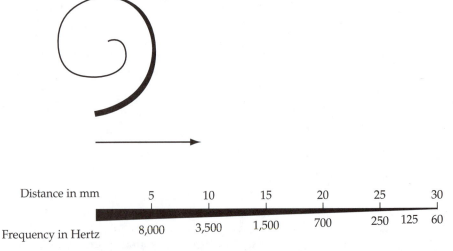

FIGURE 11.1   Schematic drawing of the tonotopic organization of the cochlea. The cochlea has been "unwound" and laid out flat. The measures on top are the distance in millimeters, while the approximate frequency positions are labeled below. (Adapted from Zemlin, 1998)

The *hair cells,* which transduce the mechanical impulses of the ear into the electrical impulses that are sent to the brain, are found on the basilar membrane. What is important to realize is that the cochlea performs a type of Fourier analysis on the speech signal (Delgutte, 1980), such that many important characteristics of speech are already present in the electrical signals conveyed to the brain. For example, as we have discussed in chapter 6 on resonance, a Fourier analysis will reveal the formant frequencies, which are the relevant acoustic properties that distinguish the various vowels. Thus, it appears that the cochlea already reacts to the formant frequencies of speech.

Hint to Students

The cochlea uncovers the F_1, F_2 patterns that distinguish the various vowels.

Thus, in some ways, the ear is already capable of extracting many of the relevant acoustic properties of speech before this signal is sent to the brain. Clearly though, the brain is where the auditory signal is transformed into speech, as the complex auditory patterns of speech are matched with the appropriate words of the listener's native language. The fact that most dichotic presentations of speech stimuli result in a right ear advantage because of the left hemisphere's advantage for processing speech also serves to underscore this point. (Chapter 12 discusses dichotic listening.)

While researchers have gained a rather detailed understanding of the hearing portion of speech perception, only sketchy information is available on the neural portion of this process. Even though much detailed information is available on hearing, there are some processes that are still not clearly understood. For example, we know that there is a process called the *auditory reflex* (or *acoustic reflex*) that apparently helps to protect our ears from sustained loud noise that can lead to permanent hearing damage. Researchers, however, are not in agreement on how the auditory reflex works. Because it takes several seconds for the auditory reflex to take place, many researchers feel that it is due to a muscular adjustment. Some feel that the auditory reflex serves to change the angle of coupling between the ossicles of the middle ear. This change serves to stiffen the chain of transmission along the ossicles and diminish the displacements. It seems that a sudden loud noise is more damaging to hearing than a comparably loud noise one was expecting. No matter how the auditory reflex works, the result is to dampen the input to the cochlea. This works like an automatic sound adjustor. In fact, there is some evidence that our own loud speech can serve to stimulate an auditory reflex!

Hint to Students

Hearing involves physical displacement of air (sound wave), of structure (tympanic membrane, ossicles), and of fluid (cochlea).

Speech Production and Hearing

We will now consider how hearing plays such an important role in speech production. One way to examine this connection is to look at cases of hearing impairment and observe the consequences on production of speech.

Children born with hearing impairment will, in most cases, experience delays in the acquisition of normal language abilities, including delays of up to two years in the acquisition of phonological, morphological, semantic, and syntactic rules. Apparently, even in the babbling stage, hearing-impaired children's babbling is qualitatively and quantitatively different from children with normal hearing (Stoel-Gammon & Otomo, 1986). The literature is contradictory, however, on whether delays in language acquisition are followed by full mastery of the native language or permanently impaired language abilities. Researchers are also uncertain how much correlation exists between the extent of hearing loss and the exact degree of linguistic impairment.

In the normal adult language system, auditory feedback plays a role in speech production. Experiments with *delayed auditory feedback* (DAF), in which speakers hear their own voices with a delay of even less than a half-second, show that their speech typically becomes dysfluent. When auditory feedback is altered in other ways as well, filtered or changed in volume, speakers tend to alter their speech to try to compensate for the acoustic changes (e.g., Yates, 1963).

Effects of Aging

In the normal language system, aging may also affect hearing and consequently speech production and perception. Long-term hearing loss may eventually affect speech production. Even in one's twenties, distinctions between high-frequency sounds may be harder to detect. Later in life, even lower frequency distinctions may become more difficult to notice. It may be especially difficult for older people to follow a conversation in a noisy room or with some type of competing auditory stimuli such as a television or radio. One of the simplest means of compensating for less sensitive hearing is to reduce the distance between speaker and listener.

Gates and colleagues (Gates, Cooper, Kannel, & Miller, 1990) followed a group of older adults who were in their sixties, seventies, eighties, and nineties. Over 1500 people were examined and tested for such hearing skills as word recognition and the discrimination and identification of speech sounds of various intensities. While these older listeners demonstrated a reduction in all of these abilities, the researchers resisted attributing the observed losses to the aging process alone. In their opinion, at least three conditions contribute to hearing problems in the elderly: (1) normal aging, (2) long-term exposure to environmental noise, and (3) the consequences of various diseases.

It is interesting to consider that Gates and colleagues estimated that 75 percent of the subjects in their study could benefit from the use of hearing aids but had never obtained them. Many older persons deny their loss of hearing and may attempt to compensate in other ways.

Cochlear Implants

The last two decades have seen a great increase in the use of another type of device used to supplement (or even replace) hearing—the *cochlear implant*. There are two parts to a cochlear implant: a thin electrode that is surgically inserted along the cochlea and a transmitter, worn behind the ear, that transmits speech signals to the cochlear stimulator. These days the electrode inserted into the cochlea has many stimulator sites, 32 or more. They are arranged in order of frequency to reproduce the tonotopic (frequency selectivity) properties of the ear. The speech processor and transmitter are worn on the outside of the ear and are typically held in place by magnets. This device acts like an antenna to capture speech sounds and change them into radio signals that are then sent through the skin to the cochlear stimulator. Of course, the degree of hearing improvement is dependent both on the accuracy of the speech processor in capturing the important frequency distinctions of speech, the ability of the stimulator to replace the electrical stimulation of the dead or missing nerve cells in the cochlea, and the quality of the training given after the implant has been fitted. The accuracy of the stimulator is directly related to the number of stimulator sites. Although many older individuals also claim to have benefited from cochlear implants, the use of such devices is most popular in young children who were either born with profound sensorineural hearing impairment or sustained such a loss early in life. The popularity of cochlear implants has increased despite the fact that some members of the Deaf community oppose the practice of surgically implanted devices to integrate individuals into the aural-oral world.

Dorman and colleagues (Dorman, Smith, McCandless, Dunnavanti, Parkin, & Dankowski, 1990) report that individuals with one brand of cochlear implant could be categorized into excellent, above-average, and average users, and that all implanted individuals benefited to some degree, perceiving wider ranges of frequency with, than without, the device. There was also improvement in perception of certain speech sounds such as the fricatives, which rely on high frequencies for their distinguishing characteristics.

It should be pointed out that attempting to improve speech perception and speech production in individuals with hearing impairment requires a joint effort between audiologists and speech-language pathologists. While the audiologist has a greater role in the assessment and augmentation of hearing, the role of the SLP in using improved hearing for better perception of speech and in improving speech production cannot be underestimated.

Interested readers will find a growing body of research on cochlear implants and other advances in hearing aids such as digital and programmable devices. It is important to demonstrate that the cost of technological improvements is justified by real improvements in speech perception.

In our next chapter, speech perception (the second part of the hearing process) will be considered.

Study Questions

1. Without looking back at the chapter, name the parts of the outer, middle, and inner ear that were discussed.

2. It can be said that hearing is the product of converted energy. Explain.

3. What are some consequences of hearing impairment on the acquisition of language?

References

Delgutte, B. (1980). Representation of speech-like sounds in the discharge patterns of auditory-nerve fibers. *Journal of the Acoustical Society of America, 68(3)*, 843–857.

Dorman, M., Smith, L., McCandless, G., Dunnavanti, G., Parkin, J., & Dankowski, K. (1990). Pitch scaling and speech understanding by patients who use the Ineraid cochlear implant. *Ear and Hearing, 11*, 310–315.

Gates, G., Cooper, J., Kannel, W., & Miller, N. (1990). Hearing in the elderly: The Framingham cohort, 1983–1985. *Ear and Hearing, 11*, 247–256.

Stoel-Gammon, C., & Otomo, K. (1986). Babbling development of hearing-impaired and normally hearing subjects. *Journal of Speech and Hearing Disorders, 51*, 33–41.

Yates, A. (1963). Delayed auditory feedback. *Psychological Bulletin, 60*, 213–232.

Zemlin, W. (1998). *Speech and hearing science* (4th ed.) Boston: Allyn & Bacon.

12 Speech Perception

We have mainly been concerned with the *production* of speech in this book thus far. While speech production is the more visible side of speech, a speech act has not occurred until a listener has perceived the spoken speech message. We can see the lips moving and we can feel the vocal folds vibrating, but we usually do not have any outward sign that speech perception is taking place. Yet many speech disorders treated by SLPs are recognized to include a problem in speech perception. Thus, not even an introductory text on speech science should overlook speech perception.

Although speech perception is difficult to explain and comprehend, most of the time we perceive speech effortlessly. In fact, many more people in the world perceive speech than learn to read. Although many of us can learn to read written language very quickly, most listeners can comprehend speech at faster rates than they can read. In fact, most of us find it more effortful to read than to listen to speech; hence the recent popularity of audio versions of books.

It is interesting to consider how often extraterrestials are usually portrayed in American films and television as speaking and understanding English. These alien beings might not even have mouths or breath air, but they are somehow able to produce human speech. The likely reason for this is not to be found in the aliens, but rather in their human audience who tires quickly of reading subtitles!

While we will consider speech perception in this chapter, our treatment will be brief and somewhat superficial. (A more detailed consideration of speech perception can be found in Ryalls, 1996.) We hope here to sensitize future SLPs to the speech perception process. Students of speech science should realize that perceiving speech is more complex than simply "hearing" a simple tone, for example. First of all, as we have seen, speech sounds are much more complex than a simple frequency. Since speech sounds are more acoustically complex, they require more complex processing for their perception.

Speech Perception and the Acoustic Signal

It used to be thought that speech perception was entirely dependent on the acoustic signal. However, it is now recognized that listeners are constantly attempting to make linguistic sense of the acoustic signal. Listeners tend to perceive speech in ways that are semantically meaningful. In a perception experiment in which certain speech sounds have been replaced with silence, listeners tend to "replace" these missing sounds to perceive whole words (Dorman, Raphael, & Liberman, 1979). This experimental procedure is known as *phonemic restoration* in recognition of the fact that listeners tended to replace missing phonemes. In fact, many times listeners were not even aware that there was something missing from the acoustic signal! In another experiment, Strange and colleagues (Strange, Verbrugge, Shankweiler, & Edman, 1976) showed that a particular vowel with specific F_1 and F_2 values was perceived differently, depending on the sentence frame in which it was presented. Such experiments provide convincing evidence that speech perception does not depend directly upon the acoustic signal, but rather that the acoustic signal captured by our ears is processed further once it arrives in the brain. Such experiments have also led to discussion of whether speech perception is a bottom-up or a top-down process.

Proceeding from the acoustic signal to the verbal message is referred to as "bottom-up" processing, while the direction from the verbal message to the acoustic signal is known as "top-down" processing. These two can be distinguished if you think of the acoustic signal as the first thing that arrives to our ears. In other words, the acoustic signal is at the basis or "bottom" of speech perception and, as listeners, we are working "up" to a meaning. Phenomena like phonemic restoration, however, suggest a more holistic, top-down component to speech recognition, which takes context and listener expectations into consideration.

Hint to Students

A top-down approach to speech perception claims that other information, such as context, is considered prior to the processing of acoustic cues to speech segments.

Categorical Perception

One speech perception phenomenon that is important for SLPs and audiologists is *categorical perception*. Categorical perception represents one of the ways in which speech is thought to be "special." That is, speech appears to be processed in a different manner from other auditory signals. While there is usually a very large discrepancy between the number of auditory signals that can reliably be discriminated and identified, in categorically perceived speech sounds listeners can only reliably identify about as many sounds as they can discriminate. Let's take an example. If listeners were presented different notes of the musical scale, most listeners could discriminate (hear the difference between) many more notes than they could reliably identify (recognize and label a note, such as "High C"). Liberman, Cooper, Shankweiler, and Studdert-Kennedy (1967) have estimated that a typical human listener can discriminate as many as 1200 different frequency differences, but can reliably only identify about 7! However, for speech sounds such as the contrast between voiced and voiceless stop consonants, listeners can only discriminate as many acoustic differences as they can identify or label. When listeners are presented with small differences along an acoustic dimension such as voice onset time (VOT, refer to chapter 9), they are typically not aware of small differences between various stimuli. They only seem to hear the broad differences in category. This lack of sensitivity to differences within the category is characteristic of categorical perception. For example, listeners only tend to hear voiced and voiceless consonants and not the small differences along the voicing continuum. This is one of the ways in which speech is thought to be different from other auditory signals such as musical notes.

Research with young infants has shown that humans demonstrate categorical perception at a very young age (Eimas, Siqueland, Jusczyk, & Vigorito, 1971). Many researchers interpret these results as evidence that the human perceptual system is already adapted for speech perception from birth. In other words, many believe that certain aspects of speech perception are innate or genetically determined.

Dichotic Listening Effect

Another way in which speech seems to be different from many other auditory stimuli is seen in the dichotic listening effect. The dichotic listening effect is observed when conflicting auditory speech signals are presented at the same intensity to both ears simultaneously; the right ear typically reveals significantly better performance than the left ear for verbal stimuli. In other words, listeners are typically more accurate at reporting language-based stimuli presented to their right ear than to their left ear and they often will report such right ear stimuli before left ear stimuli.

The explanation for this effect is that for most human listeners there are typically stronger contralateral (i.e., the brain hemisphere on the opposite side) connections from ear to brain than there are ipsilateral (i.e., the brain hemisphere on the same side as the ear) connections. This suggests that the left hemisphere has become specialized for processing at least some aspects of the speech signal such as is found in stop consonants and whole syllables.

Vowel speech signals do not typically reveal consistent ear effects in dichotic presentation, which suggests that they are less dependent on the specialized auditory processing that seems to be located in the left hemisphere in most listeners. This is possible given a vowel's more gradual onset and longer "steady-state" nature. That is, the acoustic information that specifies vowel sounds does not change as quickly as the acoustic information which specifies stop consonants. However, it is also possible that some listeners have language-processing abilities located in the right hemisphere, a situation that occurs more often in the case of left-handers. While most left-handers still have specialized speech processing located in the left hemisphere, there are more individuals with speech centers in the right hemisphere than there are among right-handers.

Hint to Students

The encoded nature of speech sounds, that is, overlapping and redundant cues, seems to go hand-in-hand with such phenomena as categorical perception and the dichotic listening effect, facilitating rapid and accurate recognition of speech. Vowles and nonspeech sounds, found to be less encoded, do not seem to be perceived categorically, nor do they show the dichotic listening effect that consonants and full syllables show.

The belief, then, that speech is a special type of auditory signal is based on the observation that speech signals can result in categorical perception and right-ear effects in dichotic listening, which are not observed with other non-speech auditory signals.

Although speech synthesis has improved over the years so that artificial speech can sound more natural than the robotic sounds of old sci-fi movies, it is much more difficult to create computer programs that recognize speech with the accuracy of a human listener. (A colleague of ours worked on such a project in the 1980s, and reported that his computer perceived the phrase "recognize speech" as "wreck a nice beach." To tell the truth, even the human perceptual system can mishear speech.) We need to learn even more about the human perceptual system, such as whether there exist invariant cues to each speech sound, regardless of context or speaker. Why is an [i] accurately recognized in all phonetic environments, and why do the [i] productions of many different people—with different fundamental frequencies and vocal tract sizes—"sound" the same? Research continues on the subject of acoustic invariance. (See Blumstein & Stevens, 1981, for further discussion.)

Importance of Mechanisms of Speech Perception

Understanding the mechanisms of speech perception is crucial to the practicing SLP. For example, the work of Paula Tallal and colleagues has examined the possibility of a central auditory processing disorder (CAPD) at the core of many cases of language-learning impaired children. Not all researchers are in agreement, but many contend that CAPD only affects speech sounds and does not affect the normal processing of less acoustically complex auditory signals such as sounds of the environment. Tallal and researchers (Tallal, Miller, Bedi, Byma, Wang, et al.,1996) claim to have developed an effective method for improving speech perception among children with CAPD. This treatment consists of specialized auditory training, in a video game-like format, in which the more acoustically complex aspects of the speech signal (i.e., the formant transitions) are first artificially increased in duration and volume, and then gradually returned to normal durations as the child's perceptual skills improve.

Notice that the aspect of the speech signal that is altered—emphasized—corresponds to the "encoded" portion of speech, where cues to several speech segments can be found. In the formant transitions from [b] to [a] in the syllable [ba], for example, the transitional area offers acoustic cues to both the stop consonant and the vowel.

This is just one of the areas in which considerable advancement in speech language pathology is being made through an increased consideration of speech perception. The attention to speech perception is likely to gain momentum in speech language pathology over the next decade.

In chapter 13, we move on to a discussion of *neurolinguistics*, an interdisciplinary field of science that explores the neural mapping of language structures and functions.

Study Questions

1. How are consonants and vowels processed differently from nonspeech auditory stimuli?

2. What similarities might there be between vowels and musical stimuli?

3. What is categorical perception and how does it facilitate speech recognition?

4. How does the treatment of CAPD that was discussed above reinforce the concept that "speech is special"?

References

Blumstein, S., & Stevens, K. (1981). Phonetic features and acoustic invariance for speech. *Cognition, 10,* 25–32.

Dorman, M., Raphael, L., & Liberman, A. (1979). Some experiments on the sound of silence in phonetic perception. *Journal of the Acoustical Society of America, 65,* 1518–1532.

Eimas, P., Siqueland, E., Jusczyk, P., & Vigorito, J. (1971). Speech perception in infants. *Science, 171,* 303–306.

Liberman, A., Cooper, F., Shankweiler, D., & Studdert-Kennedy, M. (1967). Perception of the speech code. *Psychological Review, 74,* 431–461.

Ryalls, J. (1996). *A basic introduction to speech perception.* San Diego, CA: Singular.

Strange, W., Verbrugge, R., Shankweiler, D., & Edman, T. (1976). Consonant environment specifies vowel identification. *Journal of the Acoustical Society of America, 60,* 213–221.

Tallal, P., Miller, S., Bedi, G., Byma, G., Wang, X., Nagarajan, S., Schreiner, C., Jenkins, W., & Merzenich, M. (1996). Language comprehension in language-learning impaired children improved with acoustically modified speech. *Science, 271,* 81–84.

CHAPTER

13 Neurolinguistics

Recent years have seen the growth of a subfield of linguistics, neurolinguistics, which is specifically concerned with the issues of brain-language connections. This chapter will explore neurolinguistics from several perspectives. We will examine the neurology involved in the production of speech. Then we will turn to the issue of speech perception and the associated neural areas.

Neurological Background

To start, a brief review of some basic neurology is in order. We will begin with larger structures. The human brain consists of two *hemispheres* connected by a bundle of fibers called the *corpus callosum*, allowing the right and left hemispheres to communicate with each other and to integrate information. Our brains can also be seen in terms of layers within each hemisphere. The uppermost layer is the *neocortex* (neo=new). Underneath is the *limbic system* or *paleo-mammalian section*, a layer of neuronal matter found in other species. (A brief comparison of human and non-human primate neurology will follow in chapter 14.) The deepest level, the *reptilian layer*, includes such subcortical structures as the *basal ganglia*, generally involved in regulating voluntary movement. In a general manner, older and more basic functions are found in the deeper "older" areas of the brain, while more uniquely human functions rely on the newer, more superficial neocortex. But this is more of a general tendency than a strict rule. The brain is, ultimately, a system with an integration of information across levels.

Finally, within each hemisphere, the brain can be subdivided into four areas called lobes: (1) the *frontal lobe,* which controls motor functions; (2) the *temporal lobe,* which controls auditory functions; (3) the *occipital lobe,* which is associated with vision; and (4) the *parietal lobe,* which is involved in the integration of sensory information. The frontal lobe is divided from the parietal lobe by the *central sulcus,* also known as the *Rolandic fissure*; while the temporal lobe is divided from the frontal lobe by the *Sylvian fissure.* Below the parieto-occipital area lies a structure called the *cerebellum,* which helps execute sequential maneuvers, as well as helps to control smooth voluntary movement. The lobes and these important neural land-marks are illustrated in Figure 13.1.

The articulators and other structures involved in the production of speech will be examined next with reference to neural control.

Speech Production

Cases of specific language impairments associated with injuries to the cortex (cortical insult) started appearing in the medical journals of the last century. These findings led to the emergence of neurolinguistics as a discipline that attempted to provide an answer to the question of where and how language is represented in the human brain. One of the most important discoveries of the nineteenth century can largely be credited to the founding French neuropsychologist Paul Broca. In 1861, Broca published a report in the *Bulletins de la Société Anatomique de Paris.* Although there had been discussion at the meetings of the Anatomical Society that the frontal lobes were more important for language than the more posterior portions of the brain, Broca found that it was the left frontal lobe that was particularly responsible for what he called "articulate language." Broca based his hypothesis on a clinical case—a man known by the only word he could utter—Tan. Tan had for a number of years the serious language and speech problems we now know as aphasia.

Broca's patient passed away and Broca had the opportunity to study the patient's brain upon autopsy. This was the only method scientists had at that time

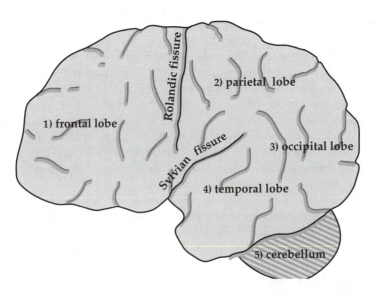

FIGURE 13.1   Schematic diagram illustrating the location of the Rolandic and Sylvian fissures and other neural landmarks of the brain.

for viewing the brain. It was a good fifty years before neurologists were able to image the brain by X-ray and nearly a century before the CAT scan (which stands for computerized axial tomography). Today, there are even more modern methods available for imaging the brain such as PET scan (positron emission tomography), SPECT (single photon emission computed tomography), and the non-radiation based MRI (magnetic resonance imaging). Broca's method of carefully observing the brain upon autopsy was the method that laid the basic foundations of modern neuropsychology.

When Broca observed Tan's brain, there was a rather large area of damage concentrated in the anterior portion of the left hemisphere. Although the damaged area was large, Broca deduced that only the central area was the portion of the brain that had been affected in the original stroke producing the patient's aphasia. This area of the brain later came to be known as *Broca's area*. Figure 13.2 illustrates Broca's area.

Two years later, Broca published another important article on aphasia. In this article, Broca presents ten additional cases supporting his hypothesis that it is the anterior portion of the left hemisphere that is especially important for articulate speech. It is ironic that Broca actually called the disorder "aphemia" and that the disorder that is named after him is actually a term advocated by Trousseau, a contemporary of Broca (Ryalls, 1984). In this second article, Broca speculates further that it is especially the "third frontal convolution" (a convolution is a ridge or mound of tissue on the surface of the brain) that is responsible for language production (Ryalls & Lecours, 1996).

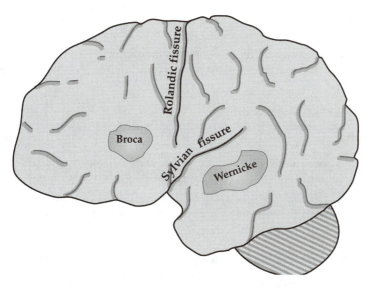

FIGURE 13.2   Schematic diagram illustrating the approximate location of Broca's and Wernicke's areas in the left cerebral hemisphere.

The frontal lobe is situated near the motor strip, an area controlling the movement of the articulators and other speech muscles. A specific region in this lobe, Broca's area has been implicated in the control of articulation and, most recently, syntactic abilities (Lieberman, 1991). Data suggest that production of speech sounds, morphologically complex words, and syntactically correct sentences are controlled by Broca's area.

Hint to Students

The following terms are somewhat equivalent in the literature on aphasia: Broca's aphasia, nonfluent aphasia, agrammatic aphasia, and predominantly expressive aphasia.

Effortful, agrammatic speech is often associated with damage in Broca's area. Lieberman (1991) points out that the existence of Broca's area is not exclusive to humans, but only in our neurology is it associated with vocalization. The frontal lobe near the motor strip is associated with skilled, coordinated manual movements. This motor control may well be the foundation for grammar: precise ordering of elements and the comprehension of such ordering and reordering of basic units of language. Human speech is *encoded*, in that the acoustic and articulatory properties of speech sounds are not isolated but rather influence neighboring segments, both prior and subsequently (encoding is also discussed in chapter 12). *Strewn*, for example, contains the rounded vowel [u]. In production, the rounding shows up three segments early, for the consonant cluster [str] is produced with protruded lips. In addition, the vowel is followed by a nasal consonant, and in English the nasal cavity tends to open in anticipation of an upcoming nasal segment while still in production for a vowel, resulting in a nasalized vowel sound.

Hint to Students

Broca's area is not synonymous with the motor cortex. Some individuals exhibit motor impairment (dysarthria) without the language or speech disorders associated with Broca's aphasia.

This encoding allows for rapid articulation, redundant clues to ensure better comprehension of speech, and a way to combat human short-term memory limitations. Lieberman (1991) claims that these complex movements of articulation, once learned, become automatized, hard-wired into the neural network. Indeed, his discussion of syntax as an automatized routine with precise ordering of elements goes on to claim that syntax is the one language ability that separates humans from all other species. Further, syntax is said to be separable from motor control.

Hint to Students

Although aphasia has tended to be associated with an interruption of speaking abilities, all modalities are vulnerable to impairment: comprehension of spoken and written language as well as the ability to write, take dictation, and initiate speech.

Naming is another linguistic component that neurolinguists have tried to map onto cerebral structures. It appears that the ability to name and to learn to associate label to meaning may be represented throughout the brain. *Anomia*, the loss of naming ability, is seen in the presence of many types of cerebral injuries. In addition, naming need not even be represented in the neocortex, because chimps, dolphins, and even dogs can be taught to associate label and meaning. (But note that it is controversial to define naming in terms of associative learning.)

How words are accessed from the mental dictionary (mental lexicon) that we all possess has been studied with considerable interest by linguists. There is evidence that words are organized and activated in semantic fields, sets of similar meanings clustered together. When you say *brother*, for example, other relationship words in the vicinity are primed, that is, activated, for example, *sister*, *son*. Another belief is that words are stored by phonological similarity, so that *brother* may be stored near *bother* and *broth*.

Hint to Students

No matter how linguists believe words are represented mentally, we all have personal, connotative meanings to words. For one of the authors, the word *Boston* brings to mind the word *jeans*, because that's where she bought her most favorite pair of jeans.

Not long after Broca's pioneering work on aphasia in France, Carl Wernicke, working in Germany, discovered another type of aphasia that would later be associated with his name (Wernicke, 1908). While damage to the anterior portion of the left hemisphere (i.e., Broca's area) typically produces more of a motor speech problem in most adults, damage to the posterior portion of the left hemisphere usually results in more of a language-level disturbance. Figure 13.2 illustrates the location of Wernicke's area.

Patients with Wernicke's aphasia do not usually have any difficulty with fluent speech production. However, there may be many errors present in this fluent speech. Sometimes, there are so many errors that the speech is not recognizable as English and is known as *jargon*. Words that are not recognizable words of a language are known as *neologisms* (equivalent to *new words*). Such patients do not typically have good comprehension, and they may even try to blame their difficulty in communicating upon the listener. They may suffer from *agnosia*, a denial of their illness. Broca's aphasics, in contrast, tend to have preserved comprehension, despite their extreme difficulty in producing fluent speech.

Studies of aphasic patients' repeated attempts to produce a particular word have shown that Broca's aphasics tend to get closer to their intended targets with each attempt, while Wernicke's aphasics tend to get further from the intended target with each try (Joanette, Keller, & Lecours, 1980). Another indication that Broca's aphasics have preserved comprehension is that they have a tendency to correct themselves, and they are apparently often very frustrated by their difficulty in producing fluent speech. More discussion of language disorders stemming from brain injury can be found in chapter 16.

Hint to Students

In the literature on aphasia the following terms are largely equivalent: Wernicke's aphasia, fluent aphasia, posterior aphasia, sensory aphasia, jargon aphasia, and predominantly receptive aphasia.

Although we have completed a very quick overview of the beginnings of modern human neuropsychology, we have also laid out some of the most important basic findings relating language function to particular areas of the brain. The first finding is that, in most adults, the left hemisphere of the brain is more crucial to language functioning than is the right hemisphere of the brain. It is also believed, however, that people who are left-handed have a greater tendency than right-handers to have speech and language localized in the opposite hemisphere (i.e., the right hemisphere). However, there is not as great a difference between left- and right-handers as seems to be commonly believed. While approximately 95 percent of right-handers have speech and language localized to the left hemisphere of the brain, the figure for left-handers is about 75 percent. Although this is a sizable reduction, supporting the notion that handedness has a neurological impact in most humans, it is important to emphasize that the majority of left handers have speech and language in the left hemisphere—just as right-handers do.

Another important principle of neurolinguistics is that, although they do not look any different from viewing the surface of the brain, the portion of the brain *anterior* to the Rolandic fissure (or central sulcus) performs a very different function than the portion of the brain *posterior* to this important landmark in the brain. We know these areas subsume very different functions because of the extreme differences in the type of aphasia that results from damage to each of these respective areas.

In one account of the neural planning of speech, the sound units to be produced are apparently selected or chosen in Wernicke's area of the left hemisphere, where this information is transferred to Broca's area, which appears to be responsible for organizing the speech motor activity for speaking a particular word or phrase. Most researchers who believe in this particular model of brain specialization also feel that it is the *arcuate fasciculus* that serves to convey the organization from Wernicke's area to Broca's area for motor execution. This model is an outgrowth of Geschwind's work on disconnection syndromes in man (1965), which states that a disconnection of neural sites best explains language disorders. In this model, many disorders are traced to a disassociation between planning and execution.

Hint to Students

The disconnection model of language impairment states that separate areas of the brain need to connect up in order to communicate. A severing of such connections results in a language disturbance. This model also posits a serial, step-by-step organization to speech processing.

Although Geschwind's model appears to be one of the more cited, certainly some research has produced results that are inconsistent with it. For example, even though Wernicke's aphasia is thought largely to affect speech planning at the phonemic level, some studies have uncovered subtle phonetic-level differences in speech produced by Wernicke's aphasics that would not be expected from the classic model (Baum, Blumstein, Naeser, & Palumbo, 1990; Ryalls, 1984).

Some neuropsychologists have attempted to articulate a somewhat different view of the neural representation for speech. One particularly intriguing divergent model is that of Jason Brown (1977). Brown holds that the phonemic planning stage and phonetic organization portions of speech production are in fact linked at all stages of their processing. This model can be viewed as more of a parallel model because both levels are processed simultaneously, rather than the classic serial model that posits that processing from one level must be completed before the information is conveyed to Broca's area for motor speech planing. (The difference between phonemic and phonetic levels was discussed in chapter 7.)

Hint to Students

A parallel processing model of language, such as Brown's, may rely less on a localizationist picture of neurolinguistics, whereby separate parts of the brain function in isolation on separate levels of language, until the task is completed.

In addition to the four lobes of the brain and Broca's and Wernicke's areas, two other important centers of the brain should also be considered. These are the *auditory cortex* and the more specialized *Heschel's gyrus* within the larger auditory cortex. While both of these areas are apparently important in the processing for speech, we will not go into detail on their exact roles. Many students learn the cranial nerves involved in speech and language from courses in anatomy and physiology, and they may learn much more detailed neuroanatomy than presented here.

The right hemisphere has been traditionally labeled the "nonlanguage" side of the brain. Recently, studies have focused on what the right hemisphere *does* contribute to speech and language. The control of the emotional component of speech, nonpropositional or affective prosody, seems to reside in the right hemisphere (Ross, 1981). Yet, several studies focusing on the representation of propositional or linguistic prosody (word stress, sentence intonation) have concluded that these linguistic tasks seem to involve the left hemisphere (Behrens, 1988). Therefore, prosody may not be as lateralized to the right hemisphere to the same degree that speech and language appear to be in the left hemisphere (Ryalls & Behrens, 1988). The right hemisphere is still being explored to understand its function alone and as part of the whole neural system.

The rate at which scientists are learning about the brain has picked up pace recently as more and more sophisticated techniques for imaging the brain become available. One of the most promising techniques at the present time is magnetic resonance imaging (MRI). While MRI has been available for a number of years, it is only now rather widespread. Not only is MRI used to image the brain, but important work observing ongoing speech production is also being conducted using this technique on speech. MRI also has the distinct advantage of not exposing the patient to dangerous levels of radiation, since this technique is based on the magnetic fields of electrons. See Figure 13.3 for an example of a coronal plane MRI image. The white arrow is pointed at a white area caused by the plaques of multiple sclerosis in the cerebellum.

Two other brain imaging techniques are positron emission tomography (PET) and single photon emission computed tomography (SPECT). In these techniques the subject emits low levels of a radioactive isotope that has been used to "tag" oxygen or glucose. A computer detection system is used to display which areas of the brain are more active than others. The more active areas of the brain take up oxygen or use glucose at a faster rate. The image of the brain is first obtained while the subject is at rest. Then the image is derived while the subject performs a specific task, such as counting numbers out loud. The image of the brain at rest is then "subtracted" from the image of the brain performing a specific task. The resulting difference image is supposed to show those areas of the brain that are specific to the particular task under investigation. Next, we will consider the neural control of speech perception. See also chapter 12 for more discussion on the perception of spoken language.

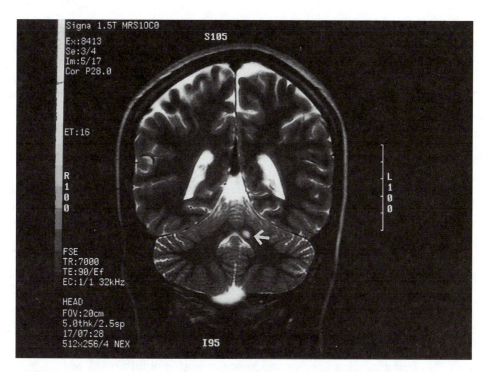

FIGURE 13.3 **Photograph of a magnetic resonance image (MRI) taken in the coronal plane. The image slice is taken 28 cm behind the anterior commissure, cutting through the parietal lobes and cerebellum. The "feathery" cerebellar cortex is evident. Subcortical matter appears much darker than the light gray and white of the cortex. Cerebrospinal fluid appears white. A white arrow points towards a bright white lesion in the cerebellum. This lesion is due to the plaques of multiple sclerosis. (Reprinted through the courtesy of Dr. Howard Chertkow, Associate Professor in the Department of Neurology and Neurosurgery, McGill University, Montreal, Canada.)**

Speech Perception

Wernicke's area lies in the temporal lobe of the left hemisphere, and while general auditory problems do not seem to arise with damage to this site, speech perception appears to suffer. Wernicke's aphasics have trouble comprehending speech at all levels: phonemically, lexically, and grammatically. General speech perception abilities, then, may be associated with the region known as Wernicke's area.

As noted earlier, Broca's region is associated with the coordination of the articulators. Little data exist to suggest any specific phonemic perception abilities associated with this area. Nonfluent aphasics seem to be well aware of their production problems and will often attempt to correct themselves.

Remember that the frontal area has been implicated in speech of a grammatical nature. Recent research has made some startling findings about the role of Broca's area in speech perception, specifically the decoding of complex syntactic structures. Damage in this region may impair an individual's ability to comprehend such syntactic structures as reversible passives and other constructions, the meanings of which hinge on function words and bound morphemes. For example, a nonreversible passive sentence such as "The flower was picked by Cathy" does not follow world knowledge if a listener attempts to process the sentence without attending to such elements as the prepositional *by* phrase and passive verb construction. In other words, even if this sentence is taken to have the structure of doer-action-receiver, real-world knowledge should cue the listener that it ultimately cannot have an active-voice meaning: In the real world flowers do not pick people.

On the other hand, "Flora was seen by Cathy" is a reversible passive, because the assignment of subject to *Flora* and to *Cathy* are both logically possible. These types of sentences cause trouble for individuals who suffer damage in Broca's area, where sentences are typically processed as active-voice utterances. These sentences cause more trouble than do nonreversible passive sentences (Caramazza & Zurif, 1976; Wulfeck, 1988).

A controversy in the field of neurolinguistics surrounds the issue of language independence from cognition. Lieberman (1991) believes that language is an overlaid function on existing cognitive structures. Hence, a language deficit will be accompanied by a cognitive loss. Naming and lexical abilities may well be preserved, but syntactic skills are affected. Lieberman points to naming as an ability found in other species and hence an earlier ability upon which speech and language are built.

Other researchers, however, claim that cognition and language are separate modules, each vulnerable to separate damage. Cases such as linguistic idiot savants and aphasics with intact intelligence are cited to prove this theory of "modularity" of functions. "Modules" are areas of the brain devoted to specific processing. However, it is beyond the scope of this text to pursue the issue of modularity in any great detail. Interested readers are referred to Fodor (1983).

In the next chapter, we look at some theories of the origins and evolution of language as well as the properties that all human languages seem to share.

Study Questions

1. What is the aim of the field of neurolinguistics?

2. What was Paul Broca's contribution to this field?

3. Explain how the concept of agrammatism has changed over time.

4. Contrast the symptoms of Broca's and Wernicke's aphasia, concentrating on the production of speech.

References

Baum, S., Blumstein, S., Naeser, M., & Palumbo, C. (1990). Temporal dimensions of consonant and vowel production: An acoustic and CT scan analysis of aphasic speech. *Brain and Language, 39,* 33–56.

Behrens, S. (1988). The role of the right hemisphere in the production of linguistic stress. *Brain and Language, 33,* 104–127.

Broca, P. (1861). Rémarques sur le siège de la faculté du language articulé suivies d'une observation d'aphemie (perte de la parole). *Bulletins de la Société Anatomique de Paris, 36,* 330–357.

Brown, J. (1977). *Mind, brain and consciousness: The neuropsychology of cognition.* New York: Academic Press.

Caramazza, A., & Zurif, E. (1976). Dissociation of algorithmic and heuristic processes in language comprehension. *Brain and Language, 3,* 572–582.

Fodor, J. (1983). *The modularity of mind.* Cambridge, MA: MIT Press.

Geschwind, N. (1965). Disconnexion syndromes in animals and man. *Brain, 88,* 237–294.

Joanette, Y., Keller, E., & Lecours, A. R. (1980). Sequences of phonemic approximations in aphasia. *Brain and Language 11,* 30–44.

Lieberman, P. (1991). *Uniquely human.* Cambridge, MA: Harvard University Press.

Ross, E. (1981). The aprosodias: Functional-anatomical organization of the affective components of language in the right hemisphere. *Archives of Neurology, 38* 561–569.

Ryalls, J. (1984). A study of vowel production in aphasia. *Brain and Language, 29,* 48–67.

Ryalls, J., & Behrens, S. (1988). An overview of changes in fundamental frequency associated with cortical insult. *Aphasiology, 2,* 107–115.

Ryalls, J., & Lecours, A. R. (1996). Broca's first two cases: From bumps on the head to cortical convolutions. In C. Code, C. Wallesche, Y. Joanette, & A. R. Lecours (Eds.), *Classic cases in neuropsychology* (pp. 235–242). East Sussex, UK: Psychology Press.

Wernicke, C. (1874). *Der aphasische symptomen-komplex.* Breslau: Cohn and Weigert.

Wulfeck, B. (1988). Grammaticality judgments and sentence comprehension in agrammatic aphasia. *Journal of Speech and Hearing Research, 31,* 72–81.

14 Evolution and Language Universals

Non-human primates are our most closely related relatives, evolutionarily as well as neurologically. While scientists cannot look directly at the development of the human brain over time, they can compare the current state of human neurology to the great apes, specifically the chimpanzee, and to the monkey.

While non-human primates have a neocortex, the function of this top layer does not match that of the human cortex. In addition, the neocortex has been "enhanced" in modern man (Lieberman, 1991). While there is an homologous Broca's area in the other primates, this area does not seem to control vocalization and movement of articulators. Instead, a subcortical area called the *cingulate cortex* in primates appears to activate vocalization when stimulated in experiments. The components of neurology associated with humans that are found in less developed forms in non-humans are called "evolutionary add-ons" by Lieberman.

The overlaying of new functions on preexisting structures is his view of how evolution exploited equipment already present and enhanced it to allow for a species with speech and language abilities.

Mentalese

Pinker (1994), in his latest interpretation of Chomsky's work, states that since all members of the human species share the same basic neurology, it stands to reason that there would be some types of universal properties shared by all languages. Certain theories even question a fundamental property of language: the arbitrary and language-specific pairing of sound and meaning (i.e., naming).

Sound symbolism, also known as *phonetic symbolism*, posits a psychological correlate to the phonetic structure of languages. For example, it appears that words signifying small objects in many languages contain the sound ee (/i/), which in articulatory terms is produced with the tongue very high and front in the mouth. In other words, the oral cavity forward of the tongue position is small, and there may be some mental connection between small objects and small oral space. In English, words such as *teeny, mini,* and the diminutive suffix *-y* (Tommy, Johnny, Susy) refer to a smallness.

In addition, words (in English, anyway) beginning with the consonant blend "sl" tend to have associations in people's minds with low-friction qualities: for example, slimy, slick, slippery, and slither. (Can you name others? And some counter examples?) Some people claim that there is a natural association between colors and sounds, such as between primary colors and vowel sounds (Ryalls, 1983).

While linguistics has come a long way towards accepting the similarities of languages and deemphasizing differences, phonetic symbolism as a theory of mind determining language has not won many followers. *Mentalese* is a recent term used to define the language that humans think in. Many researchers would disagree with a claim that English speakers "think" in English, Spanish speakers in Spanish, and so on. Mentalese is an idea that has replaced for many the theory of linguistic determinism, which we will now discuss.

Linguistic Determinism

Work done in the early part of the twentieth century by Edward Sapir and his student Benjamin Whorf assumed a deterministic connection between the specific language one speaks and the state of that individual's cognition. The *Sapir-Whorf Hypothesis*, as their theory became known, claims that language molds and shapes thinking. If your language does not have specific color terms for different shades of blue and green, for example, and you label all these hues as "green," cognitively they *are* all one color to you.

Whorf concentrated on Native American languages and published "facts" claiming that Navajo speakers cannot discriminate blue from green since both colors are subsumed under one label. Other claims were made about Apache, Hopi, and even Chinese and Eskimo languages (Whorf, 1956).

Criticism, however, soon rained down on the Sapir-Whorf Hypothesis, with good reason. For starters, Whorf's translations of non-English languages were inaccurate. Clumsy translations cannot determine much. Secondly, the Sapir-Whorf Hypothesis focused a great deal on grammar. Grammar alone is not language, nor is grammar the same thing as cognition. Other flaws in the Sapir-Whorf data soon weakened the persuasiveness of linguistic determinism (although the folk legend that Eskimos have an igloo-full of words for snow continues to make the rounds in spite of being debunked [Pullum, 1991]).

A weaker version of linguistic determinism, *linguistic relativism*, surfaces in discussions of "sexist" language and is behind such linguistic innovations as *s/he* and the spelling revision in *womyn*. Male-dominated terms, the reasoning goes, sustain a male-dominated society; others argue that they merely reflect the social structure or even have no bearing on society. The situation is not a simple one, and the argument continues.

Universal Grammar

Another way language studies have changed since the Sapir-Whorf Hypothesis is in the acknowledgment of, and search for, so-called language universals predicted by Pinker's statement above. While Sapir and Whorf concentrated on language differences, popular in the early century, Chomsky and others starting in the late 1950s began discussions of a *Universal Grammar* and the language aspects that all languages share. These universals can be shared elements, called *substantive universals*; they can also be universals of form (*formative universals*), which entail the rules that order certain elements.

After a cursory reading of the literature on language universals, one is impressed with the degree of similarity among the world's languages. Yet the initial reaction one has when confronting a speaker of a "foreign" language is the inability to communicate. The lack of mutual intelligibility is what we notice first and emphasize. Linguists have been at work, however, on documenting the similarities on other levels besides vocabulary.

Absolute Universals

All human languages start with a small set of building blocks, *phonemes*, that can be combined in various ways to produce a much wider pool of words and an indefinite number of sentences. This characteristic of language would be classified under the term *absolute universals*, along with such other properties common to all known languages as making use of consonants and vowels, differentiating between nouns and verbs, and allowing the transformation of sentences into interrogatives and negations.

Statistical Universals

Absolute universals are the rarest of the language universal types. There are also properties that appear in *most* languages, but not all. They are termed *statistical universals*. Most known languages, for example, follow a subject-object-verb (SOV) word order (Japanese, Korean) or a subject-verb-object (SVO) order (English). While verb-subject-object (VSO) and other arrangements are known, they are much less common. Therefore, SOV and SVO are word orders that can be classified as statistical universals.

Unrestricted Universals

Another way to categorize universals is in terms of their independence from any other element in the language. Universals whose existence is independent of other occurrences in the language are called unrestricted universals.

Implicational Universals

An element or rule contingent upon the existence of another element or rule is an *implicational universal*. Implicational universals can be thought of in an "if x, then y" arrangement; often they occur in series called *implicational chains*. For example, if a language has indirect objects, then it will also have direct objects. Direct objects, consequently, signal the existence of agents (subjects). In this way, a chain of implications arises, but only unidirectionally: If a language has direct objects, it need not also have indirect ones (Aitchison, 1996).

With the examination of universals, one can see that languages don't simply "do what they want," that is, vary in completely random and unpredictable ways. While all languages change, they tend to change in relatively unsurprising ways and never lose their systematicity.

Constraints on Language (Filters)

Another factor that can explain the regularity of languages is that human language has *constraints* placed upon it. We don't mean the grammar school warnings about double negatives and split infinitives. There exist very real boundaries that contain language. One type involves physical limits: Languages don't make use of speech sounds that cannot be perceived by the human auditory system, or sounds that are extremely difficult to produce, such as a stop with a very long VOT lead. Nor would sentences that tax the short-term memory of speaker and listener alike be tolerated. These types of constraints are called *filters*.

Preferences

Likewise, humans have *preferences* that are reflected in the properties of language. Remember that SOV and SVO word orders were the most popular in the world's languages? We seem to have a preference for the actor (subject) to be mentioned first. Other developmental strategies are observed in children acquiring their first language, alerting linguists to the human preferences that shape individual languages. Children learning names for objects tend to prefer one label for one object (*mutual exclusivity principle*) and tend to assume that the label refers to the whole object, not just a part of it (*whole object principle*). More can be found on learning strategies and operating principles in chapter 15.

Hint to Students

Language *universals* describe what languages share. Language *filters* and language *preferences* explain why certain patterns exist.

Language Acquistion and Language Universals

One may wonder how much these linguistic constraints and universals stem from our shared anatomy, neurology, and cognitive systems. Researchers such as Lieberman claim that universals should not surprise us since language is a facility built on preexisting cognitive structures. Even linguists who believe language is in a separate "module" from cognitive skills, such as Chomsky (1980), would agree that universals can be traced to the basic wiring for language we are all born with, be it separate from cognition or not.

Finally, the question arises why infants need to develop and acquire language at all—Why aren't our young born with a full language system already in place? A related question is, Why does the language acquisition facility seem to shut off for so many of us after a certain age? Learning a new language after our childhoods can be grueling, difficult, and frustrating work, and even with concentrated effort it still may not lead to native competence in that new language.

These two questions are related in that they both involve the neurology of the human brain. According to Chomsky, we are born with a language acquisition device that contains all the wiring to make language possible. We have a predisposition to acquire a human language, and we are given a leg-up advantage with principles, strategies, and preferences. What we need is exposure to a speech community, an interactional exchange with other speakers of a language, and the time to practice. It is during this time, between birth and the acquisition of a full language system, that the child's neurology differentiates into specific language centers and the vocal tract matures and changes, allowing for a wealth of speech sounds. Before three months of age, the larynx is high in the throat, allowing the baby to drink and breathe simultaneously. This is a good set-up for survival, but it does not allow for the production of some important speech sounds, namely the vowels [u a i]. Once the larynx is lowered, the L-shaped vocal tract can produce these so-called quantal vowels. The right angle bend in the adult human vocal tract allows the tongue to separate the two distinct resonating chambers that these vowels require. The developing child also gains greater coordination over the articulators. However, the individual is now vulnerable during eating, for food can more easily enter the lungs. Some researchers view human beings' vulnerability to swallowing problems as the price we have had to pay for our ability to speak. This relationship may be viewed as support for SLPs being the health professionals most appropriate for treatment of swallowing disorders (dysphagia).

Linguists also point out that if a child were to be born speaking, what language would he or she speak, and what if it were not intelligible to the society around the child? One needs to communicate, a main function of language. Chomsky's Principles and Parameters Theory (1980) states that children are born with the principles of human language, and they also possess parameters, ways to set their developing language knowledge to the tune of the language they are exposed to. For example, the target language might be an SOV language, an SVO language, or one of the less common word order languages. The child "knows" (internally) there will be some type of ordering involved. With exposure and mental calculations, the child eventually sets the word-order switch (parameter) to the correct setting. Adults are not necessarily conscious of these parameters or their settings and so could not directly teach the child what to do.

The child needs to take in data and make guesses, hypothesizing about the character of his or her new language. As for the loss of the ease with which children seem to absorb their first language, that loss may seem "unfair" or a bad arrangement. A critical period is reached around puberty in which neurologically the language centers stabilize (an initial loss of some plasticity occurs between 6 and 8 years of age). Unlike cases of 2-year-olds experiencing left hemisphere trauma without aphasia, after the critical period, the brain is less able to adapt and reassign functions. In addition, the machinery for hypothesis-testing and mental calculations (called language acquisition) now becomes deliberate learning of rules and vocabulary. Of course, we continue to gain new lexical items and even perhaps verbal dexterity in the years after the critical period, but we do not again have the ability to use our innate wiring to acquire another language system with the same facility. There are, of course, exceptions—people "good at language" who continue to add to their linguistic repertoire throughout life; why they can is a bit of a mystery. In addition, the idea of a critical period in humans has been questioned by research into second language acquisition (see Hakuta, 1986).

Other species experience a critical period as well. The white crowned sparrow needs exposure to the song of its species by a certain age or it will never master a native-like singing (Marler, 1975). Why does a critical period exist? Neurologically, the brain is moving on to other tasks. Pinker (1994) estimates that the brain consumes 20 percent of our blood's oxygen, and the cost of maintaining a flexible language facility after the age at which one is usually set with a full system seems wasteful, kind of like keeping the furnace going in the summer. Once we reach puberty and linguistic maturity, we move on to reproduction (that is the original plan, anyway) and leave linguistic acquisition to the next generation. Cruel as it may sound, once we reproduce, we may well be less valuable to our species than are the younger members who have not yet reproduced. Keeping the species going is a large driving force in our design, and it shows in our neurological wiring.

Which brings us back to the concept of mentalese, the language we all think in. If language potential is present at birth, or perhaps even prenatally (Chomsky, 1980), that commonality all humans share may well be reflected in a shared language of thought, even after the parameters are set.

In the next two chapters, we consider the normal development of a speech production system (chapter 15) and the disorders that may arise in the production of speech (chapter 16).

Study Questions

1. Explain the different types of language universals that have been proposed.

2. Describe Chomsky's Principles and Parameters Theory.

3. What is the "mutual exclusivity principle" and how does it relate to the "whole object principle"?

4. What are language constraints and how do they operate?

References

Aitchison, J. (1996). *The seeds of speech*. Cambridge, UK: Cambridge University Press.

Chomsky, N. (1980). *Rules and representations*. New York: Columbia University Press.

Hakuta, K. (1986). *The mirror of language*. New York: Basic Books.

Lieberman, P. (1991). *Uniquely human*. Cambridge, MA: Harvard University Press.

Marler, P. (1975). On the origin of speech from animal sounds. In J. Kavanagh & J. Cutting (Eds.), *The role of speech in language* (pp. 11–37). Cambridge, MA: MIT Press.

Pinker, S. (1994). *The language instinct*. New York: William Morrow & Company.

Pullum, G. (1991). *The great Eskimo vocabulary hoax*. Chicago: University of Chicago Press.

Ryalls, J. (1983). Synesthesia: A principle for the relationship between the primary colors and the vowels. *Semiotica, 58,* 107–121.

Whorf, B. L. (1956). *Language, thought and reality: Selected writings of Benjamin Lee Whorf* (ed. J. B. Carroll). Cambridge, MA: MIT Press.

15 Development of Speech Production

A prerequisite to any course in speech pathology is the study of the normal development of speech production. Speech-language pathologists need a baseline measure of normal production to then work with pathologies. These measures include the pronunciation of speech sounds (phonetics), acquisition and use of vocabulary (lexicon and semantics), and production of grammatical markers and the organization of utterances (morphosyntactic development). Researchers also examine the development of the social functions of speech and the pragmatic skills of developing children.

We are not born speaking, but studies have shown an innate language potential in very young infants. Right from birth, children prefer to hear the sounds of speech as opposed to nonspeech sounds. In addition, they prefer the sounds of their own speech community to those of other languages. Finally, when presented with the speech of their own mothers and that of another adult female, they prefer to listen to their mothers' production (Berko Gleason, 1997).

These findings all suggest that a language potential, or instinct, is in place at birth. We will examine the development of language in normal cases at each linguistic level.

Children progress through a sequence of developmental stages that are seen across language communities. Each stage may be characterized from a phonological, lexical, morphosyntactic, and pragmatic perspective. Movement from one stage to the next may be abrupt, and the time a child remains in a particular stage can vary by individual.

Prelingual Stage (0–6 months*)

At this stage, utterances are considered nonlinguistic in nature, that is, they are nonpropositional, neither naming nor commenting on objects in the child's environment. Crying, cooing, and other nonlanguage sounds are in evidence.

---

*Ages are averages.

However, it is in this stage that infants seem to develop two important aspects of language: turn-taking abilities and native prosody. By making eye contact with adult caretakers and exchanging sound in something resembling a conversation, infants are practicing a pragmatic component of language use. In addition, the cooing evident at this early stage is by no means monotonous. As mentioned earlier, infants appear sensitive to the melody of their speech community's language. Prosodic contours on these nonlinguistic utterances seem to conform to the adult melody.

Babbling Stage (6–12 months)

At the babbling stage, the child begins to practice articulation, playing with the coordination of tongue, lips, vocal folds, and other articulators. Some researchers label this stage the *canonical babbling stage*, because syllable patterns start to emerge. Moving from the isolated vowel (V), to consonant and vowel (CV) syllables, and progressing through such syllable types as VCV, VC, and the reduplication of syllables (CVCV) and variegated syllables (e.g., /bitaku/), children start to acquire the phonemes of the language.

Researchers have traced the order in which consonants and vowels emerge, and unlike previous theories, current theory claims that not all the possible speech sounds of human language are present at the start of babbling (Locke, 1983). Some native sounds may still need to be added, while other nonnative sounds will eventually drop out.

Native prosody is in place by now, and the babbling at times may so resemble native speech that some researchers call the final month or two of this stage *conversational babbling*. Although these babbled syllables convey no semantic value, some may be *protowords*, idiosyncratic labels for objects in the child's world. Parents are sometimes not only confused by the idiosyncrasy of the labels, but the varied phonological forms these protowords can take; for example, one day *dog* is [daw] and the next it is pronounced [baw].

Consonant sounds that arrive early include anterior stops, (e.g., [p b t d]), nasal consonants (e.g., [m n]), glides (e.g., [j w]), and the two fricatives [s] and [h]. Added later are posterior stops, the remaining fricatives, the affricates, and the liquids. You may have noticed how liquids, [l r], tend to be problems for child production, with many [l] sounds substituted for [r] and vice versa—that is, glides used in place of liquids (*wabbit* for *rabbit*; one of us insisted, as a child, that the sun was the color *yeyo*). This order of acquisition, it should be remembered, is an average, with some differences found from child to child. Table 15.1 summarizes the early and later developing consonants.

The first contrast children make is between consonants and vowels, as seen in the alternating CV syllables. Later, children are aware of sounds that obstruct air flow as distinct from those that are produced with a more open vocal tract—for example, stops versus fricatives. Place contrasts seem to be made earlier than voicing distinctions. Therefore, a child may be sensitive to the bilabial/alveolar con-

TABLE 15.1   **Sequence of Developing Consonant Phonemes**

Early:

 Stops
 Nasals
 Glides
 /s/ and /h/

Later:

 Fricatives
 Affricates
 Liquids

TABLE 15.2   **Order of Sensitivity to Phonemic Features**

Consonant versus vowel
Obstruent versus continuant
Place distinctions
Voicing distinctions

trast in [b] versus [d] earlier than to the voicing distinction of [b] and [p]; children may well substitute the two bilabial sounds for each other freely, while the place distinction is respected. Consonant clusters (CC) appear later in this stage of development, first occurring utterance-initially, then later still in other positions in utterances. Table 15.2 shows the developing phonemic consonant contrasts to which children become sensitive.

Hint to Students

The child typically acquires the contrast of vowels versus consonants first, then stops versus fricatives next, and then place distinctions such as bilabial versus alveolar.

For vowels, children are more sensitive to the distinction between vowels produced with the tongue high versus low. This distinction is made earlier than that between vowels produced in the front of the oral cavity compared to farther back in the mouth. So a sensitivity to the [u]/[a] difference may develop and be available to children earlier than a difference between [u] and [i].

For languages with oral and nasal vowel phonemes, such as French, where the nasality added to a vowel produces an entirely new sound that can alter the meaning of a word, this distinction for children is typically acquired quite late. The progression of vowel contrasts that the child usually acquires, then, first is high versus low vowels, then front versus back vowels, and finally oral versus nasal vowels.

One-Word or Holophrastic Stage (1–2 years)

As protowords transition into the child's first word, he or she enters the one-word stage. This stage is also called the holophrastic stage, because one word is the equivalent of a full sentence to the child.

Hint to Students

Holo = one, phrastic = phrase or sentence — one word functions as an entire sentence.

Syllables still tend to be no more complex than the CV, VCV, or the reduplicated and variegated types seen earlier. Unlike protowords, though, the child's utterances now carry semantic meaning. In addition, these words don't simply name objects in the world; they describe and comment on objects and people.

One word may have several meanings. [daw], for *doll*, could be a request, a negation of another's utterance, a comment on an action, or a command. It could also hold a possessive meaning, as in *this is my doll*. Within the first 18 months, children concentrate on nouns, especially names of objects they have direct contact with and can interact with and change in some way. (Hence the abandonment of the old-fashioned stationary toys for the transforming, mutant ones!)

Lexical Acquisition

Language-specific labels (vocabulary) is one aspect of language that must be learned. A naming explosion around 18 months, in which the average number of words a child possesses grows from 20 to 120, has been used as evidence that children now grasp the relationship between label and object.

In fact, linguists like Slobin (1985) claim that children are born with a set of operating principles, strategies, that serve as a leg-up in the immense task of learning language-specific lexical items. First, humans are likely born with a predisposition for naming. What happens around 18 months is that the child reaches a cognitive stage when these operating principles give him or her a head start in the complex task of lexical learning.

Hint to Students

A child's meaning of a word may not be adult meaning.

Children will assume certain truths about language as they learn words. When they are presented with an object and a label—for example, *dog*—they will assume that the label is a name for the entire object and not just a part (e.g., leg, tail). This operating strategy, called the *whole object principle*, may not always result in the *correct* assumption, but it serves the child well most of the time. It also prevents lexical learning from being a process of trial and error.

Children may already have private, baby names for objects: The child of one of our students calls her blanket *binky*, while another refers to birds as *fu-fus*. Eventually, the child will realize that there is an "adult," alternative label for these objects. The *mutual exclusivity assumption* guides the child to reject the possibility of something having more than one label. The child will then settle on the name heard more frequently, the more conventional label. Thus, we see another operating principle in place, the *conventionality principle*, that resolves the conflict created by the mutual exclusivity assumption.

Children also learn to extend the meaning of words they already possess, so that small white poodles *and* large black labs will eventually both be called *dog*. This *principle of extendibility* sometimes goes too far, and cows may also be labeled *dog*, a phenomenon called *overextension* or *overgeneralization*. Mutual exclusivity and conventionality will soon alert the child to the discrepancy between his or her own label and the more common label heard in his or her environment.

Sometimes children *underextend* word meanings, so that *dog* is only a dog in a certain situation or is only a particular dog, for example, only a certain familiar dog in the park or only Snoopy sleeping on the roof of his doghouse. Again, other operating principles will eventually help the child to discover the adult meaning of words.

Finally, the *taxonomic principle* controls how extension of meaning may work. It may lead a child to extend a word's meaning to related objects but not to related actions or objects marginally related to the original object. Thus, *dog* may soon include other types of canines but may less likely be used to name the act of running in the park, sleeping on the roof of a doghouse, or the name of the dog's food-bowl (or for the food itself).

Two-Word Stage (2 years**)

By this stage, children's utterances have progressed to combinations of the three basic components of a sentence (sometimes called *thematic roles* or *sentence relationships*): agent, action, and object in the following ways, with only two roles or relationships expressed at any one time.

> agent-object [ma baw] *mommy* (action) *ball*
> agent-action [ma pu] *mommy pull* (*me*)
> action-object [pu mi] (*mommy*) *pull me*
> (Note: The implied relationship is in parentheses.)

**The estimated ages given are less reliable by this stage since there is a great deal of individual variation in how long a child remains at any one stage.

Notice that a preference for a particular word order has emerged by now. Children tend to prefer the "doer" first, especially agents that are animate or the children themselves. Clearly, the child has the concept of all these components of a subject-verb-object utterance, but he or she is not yet capable of producing all components at once. The particular meanings of these two-word utterances may vary by situation as well, so that [ma kek] (*mommy cake*) may either be a request, a command, or a statement of possession.

At the two-word stage, children build on their ability to produce negative utterances. From the previous stage, *no* was sufficient to convey negation. At this next stage, *no* placed sentence-initially can be used to negate, for example, *no pull*.

With respect to interrogatives, most languages, such as English, allow rhetorical questions, where a declarative word-order is pronounced with a rising intonation, such as *It is raining?* said with surprise. Children will start with such a device to produce question utterances and soon move on to slightly more sophisticated strategies such as adding a wh-question word to the start of an utterance, for example, *what bed*.

Content words (nouns, verbs, adjectives) are more common than function words at this stage (prepositions, conjunctions, articles).

Telegraphic Stage (MLU computed)

Utterances at this stage vary widely in length. In addition, with the absence of function words and bound morphemes (prefixes and suffixes), utterances give one the impression of listening to a telegram.

By now, researchers typically abandon chronological age and instead use a new measurement: *mean length of utterance (MLU)*. By computing each morpheme in a child's utterance and averaging across many speech samples, researchers gather an MLU count for a child.

Children at this stage lengthen the two-word sentences of the past stage in a number of ways: (1) by conjoining information, that is, using conjunctions (*Mommy and me*), (2) by adding modifiers and other phrases to expand an utterance (*big brown dog*), and (3) by using more thematic roles than before, such as adding location information to an agent-action utterance (*dog sleep on roof*). These strategies lead to what is termed *cumulative complexity*, whereby children exploit information they already possess to increase the complexity of sentences.

Hint to Students

Children expand sentences in the telegraphic stage by adding (1) conjunctions, (2) modifying words, and (3) thematic roles.

As the telegraphic stage progresses, bound morphemes and function words start to appear in children's utterances. These new parts of speech usually arrive in a predictable order (Brown, 1973), with the "-ing" suffix and prepositions such as *in* and *on* appearing early, and contractions (*Mommy's*) and helping verbs appearing late in this stage.

Let's look a little closer at one example. English morphology uses a suffix [s], [z], or [ɪz] to indicate one of the following pieces of information: plural noun, possessive, or third person singular in the present tense. Children start to utilize the "-s" ending in this order, with plurals arriving earlier than possessive markers, and the third person singular marker emerging quite late.

In addition, as children learn the language's bound morphemes (affixes), overgeneralization can arise (the same process seen in lexical learning). The regular plural rule tends to be widely applied to all nouns, regular or irregular, count or mass, with results such as *foots* and *airs*. Sometimes children will even produce *feets*; here the irregular form was originally acquired without the plural meaning and is now being pluralized like all other nouns

Children's production in this stage reflects several phonological processes in action. Actual utterances do not always match target words—for example, *time* pronounced as [daɪm]. Although it may seem this utterance is completely off target, the distinction is actually in one feature difference in one phoneme, a voicing distinction. We next examine the phonological processes involved in children's speech. Table 15.3 summarizes the stages of acquistion.

Phonological Processes

Children's production of consonants and vowels will be nearly adult-like by around 3 years of age. Problems with liquid [r, l] production may linger, and what looks like regression (an increase in errors) may occur when words are multisyllabic. In addition, some voicing distinctions may still not be produced by the child.

Certain phonological processes characterize the pronunciation of children prior to attainment of a full adult phonology. Patterns emerge in each child that can be explained by these processes.

Some phonemes tend to be replaced with other, substitute sounds. For example, the word *look* may be pronounced *wook*, in which a glide [w] replaces a liquid [l].

TABLE 15.3   Stages of Acquisition

I. Prelingual Stage (0–6 months)
II. Babbling Stage (6–12 months)
III. One-word Stage (1–2 years)
IV. Two-word Stage (approximately 2 years)
V. Telegraphic Stage (MLU computed)

This *substitution* is much more frequent than the reverse situation where a *glide* is replaced by a *liquid*. Glides tend to be mastered earlier than liquids, and we see the child avoiding a liquid here.

Another explanation for the substitution of [w] for [l] may be found. Whereas other sounds could have replaced the liquid, resulting in *yook* (another glide), *book* (a stop), or *nook* (a nasal), the [w] is closer to the target sound [l] in terms of obstruency—that is, amount of obstruction in the vocal tract during production. Glides and liquids are produced with relatively open vocal tracts compared to other manners of consonants.

We would also benefit from an examination of the entire target word. What does the substituted sound have in common with the rest of the word? [w] and [k] are both velars: They match in place of articulation. *Assimilation* is another phonological process in evidence here. Assimilation is the altering of a speech sound so that it matches more closely another sound in the phonological environment. In *wook* for *look*, initial and final consonants now match in the place feature.

Consonant cluster reduction is another phonological process we see in action in children's production of speech. Consecutive consonants are difficult for children to produce before they reach their full linguistic competence. A consonant cluster, therefore, may be reduced, and this may happen in one of two ways.

First, one of the consonants may be deleted—the specific segment being deleted is dependent on its phonological feature. *Brook*, for example, may be pronounced *book*. We have already noted that liquids are mastered quite late, and in this example, it is indeed the liquid, and not the stop consonant, that is omitted. For the word *stop*, the child might well produce /top/, and here a stop consonant is retained while a fricative is deleted.

Another way to reduce a consonant cluster is to break it apart by inserting a vowel between the two consonants. *Brook* in this case would be pronounced /barʊk/, with a vowel, usually a schwa, being added. This process of sound addition is termed *epenthesis*.

Entire words may be simplified by the child. Unstressed syllables, especially word-initial or medial, may be deleted. *Telephone*, then, would be pronounced /tɛlfon/, *recipe* would be /rɛspi/, and *alone* would be /lon/. Some words are simplified by the deletion of the final consonant, so that *spoon* may be pronounced as /pu/.

Finally, a phonological process that is seen in the babbling stage is the repetition of CV syllables. Children may *reduplicate* a CV form to pronounce a multisyllabic word. *Baba* for *baby* (or for *bottle*) and *dada* for *daddy* are such examples of reduplication. Table 15.4 summarizes the phonological processes of language development.

Now that we have reviewed the normal course of first-language development, in the next chapter we turn to the disorders associated with childhood production of language. Chapter 16 also looks at the disorders seen later in life, especially adult-onset aphasia.

TABLE 15.4 Phonological Processes of Language Development

Process	Example	
	Target Utterance	*Actual Utterance*
1. **Substitution:** One phoneme replaces another. Here, a glide substitutes for a liquid.	[lʊk]	[wʊk]
2. **Assimilation:** Alteration of phoneme to match other phoneme in the utterance. Here, initial velar sound is produced as an alveolar stop, matching the final consonant's place of articulation.	[kæt]	[tæt]
3. **Consonant-cluster reduction:**		
a) By deletion of a consonant. Here, a liquid is deleted.	[brʊk]	[bʊk]
b) By epenthesis. Here a schwa is inserted between two consonants.	[brʊk]	[barʊk]
4. **Reduplication:** Repetition of syllables. Here, CV utterance is lengthened by repetition.	[bebi]	[bababa]

Source: Adapted from Dale (1976).

Study Questions

1. What linguistic abilities are present in prelingual infants?

2. Name the five stages of speech development discussed in this chapter.

3. Assign an approximate age period to each of these stages, and briefly describe the speech characteristics of each stage.

4. Describe the learning strategies involved in first-language acquisition.

5. A friend of yours who has a young child asks your advice because she knows that you are studying to become a speech-language pathologist. Her little boy is 14 months old and still has a lot of difficulty with common words. He does not say most consonant sounds, and the vowel sounds he does use for many words are not clear enough to figure out the word he is saying. What advice would you give your friend?

References

Berko Gleason, J. (1997). *The development of language* (4th ed.). Boston: Allyn & Bacon.

Brown, R. (1973). *A first language.* Cambridge, MA: Harvard University Press.

Dale, P. S. (1976). *Language development* (2nd ed.). New York: Holt, Rinehart and Winston.

Locke, J. (1983). *Phonological acquisition and change.* New York: Academic Press.

Slobin, D. (1985). *The cross-linguistic study of language* (Volumes 1 & 2). Hillsdale, NJ: Erlbaum.

16 Disorders of Speech Production

A variety of disorders can affect the normal production of speech. We all know that we may not be as fluent as we would like speaking in front of a large audience, but fortunately this is only a temporary problem. Fatigue, stress, and overindulgence in alcohol can reveal their detrimental effects in speech production. Fortunately, these are also temporary situations. Let us consider some of the disorders that affect speech production. We will first look at production disorders more commonly found in the developing language system of children. Then we will expand our discussion to production deficits seen later in life as well.

Production Disorders in Children

We all know that young children do not speak like adults. Young children tend to simplify the pronunciation of difficult words, and these simplifications can be entertaining and even comical (one of us used to refer to *umbrellas* as *aunt brennas* and *spaghetti* was routinely called *bisketti*). Even in these simplifications we can see phonological processes at work such as *cluster reduction* and *assimilation*. Normally developing children will grow out of these simplifications when they have mastered somewhat better speech control.

Although any deviation from the development of language discussed in chapter 15 need not indicate a language problem, a variety of different disorders of speech development interfere with the normal development of speech acquisition. One of the most common of these is a slower or delayed development of speech. Probably the singlemost common cause of slower speech acquisition is abnormal hearing, and for this reason a child's hearing should be evaluated periodically throughout the developing years. Even if the possibility of permanent hearing impairment has been eliminated, young children have a higher susceptibility to middle ear infections, or otitis media, than adults. This type of ear infection can be recurrent. It is obvious that any interruption of normal hearing, even temporary, can have a detrimental effect on speech development.

Sometimes young children with delays in speech acquisition that are not due to hearing problems can make dramatic improvements and catch up with their normally developing peers. However, any child with a persistent speech delay, lasting longer than 1 year of age, should be evaluated by a professional SLP. The SLP can evaluate the child, decide whether therapy is required, initiate therapy, and oftentimes suggest exercises and activities that the parents can perform with the child at home. Many adults are very grateful for the remarkable improvement in the quality of life afforded them by the services of an SLP when they were children.

Slower development that is not due to hearing problems may have either a neurological or a muscular origin. It is typically very difficult to differentiate between the two in a precise manner. However, if the child performs other complex motor activities such as walking and coloring in a normal manner and at a typical age, the delay may be specific to speech. If this child also can perform oral motor activities such as chewing and swallowing food, imitating facial grimaces, sticking out the tongue and blowing bubbles, there is evidence that the speech delay is not simply motoric but rather more extensively neurological in nature. A speech disorder in children that is more motoric in nature may be referred to as a *dysarthria* or *dyspraxia*. Wit and colleagues have performed detailed studies of the speech performance capabilities of children with dysarthria (Wit, Maasen, Gabreels, & Thoonen, 1993).

Another aspect of childhood production disorders that has received much attention recently is *specific language impairment* or SLI. At this time there is much research attempting to define the exact etiology and manifestations of this disorder. SLI refers to language deficits that cannot be traced to problems in processing sensory information or to a disorder in general cognition. Language may be impaired at any or all linguistic levels. Specifically, function words and bound morphemes (prefixes and suffixes) may be absent. Passive sentence constructions may also be absent, as may utterances with overt subjects. Phonologically, there tend to be more instances of simplifications than in the normally developing child. Overall vocabulary may be smaller than for age-matched normal children (Cairns, 1996; Nelson, 1998).

The syndrome called *autism* also impacts the linguistic system of growing children. Overall communicative ability is severely below average. Specifically, these children may process utterances very literally, preferring concrete meanings to more abstract concepts. While syntax may appear normal, syntactic structures may be used inappropriately (e.g., a declarative used as an interrogative). Prosody may also sound inappropriate or non-native. *Echolalia* is another common trait associated with autism; it refers to the immediate or delayed repetition of utterances heard in the individual's environment (Nelson, 1998).

Production Disorders in Children and Adults

Some production disorders are not specific to childhood. We next turn to those impairments of speech production found in children and adults.

A great deal of research has gone into the disorder of *stuttering* or *dysfluency*. Yet, stuttering is still not clearly understood. However, most research into this disorder recognizes several types of contributing factors. One factor may be a problem in neuromotor timing. Some stutterers report that they feel as if the motor commands to these speech muscles are out of sync with what they are attempting to say. There is also evidence that some dysfluent speakers may actually be more fluent when the sound of their own speech is fed back to their ears with a small time delay—a condition known as *delayed auditory feedback* (DAF). However, not all stutterers can improve speech fluency with delayed auditory feedback. Very recently some work has begun to uncover a neurological basis for some types of fluency disorders. DeNil and his colleagues at the University of Toronto have shown abnormal activation patterns in PET scans of adult stutterers (DeNil, 1997). There is also some evidence that certain pharmacological agents can improve speech fluency. Although the cause and nature of stuttering is not well understood, it is fortunate that there exists a variety of effective therapy approaches to help nonfluent speakers improve their speech production. While some clients can gain rather remarkable results with relatively little therapy, other clients must invest a great deal of time and effort to improve their fluency. However, almost every client can benefit from speech-language therapy. As our understanding of this disorder improves, it is likely that more effective therapy techniques will also be developed.

A persistent speech disorder can be the result of a severe automobile or motorcycle accident. A severe injury to the head can result in *traumatic brain injury* or TBI. Although the brain is damaged, it may not be possible to locate a specific area of injury. Speech and language disorders can persist even after the patient is able to walk and perform many normal activities of daily living. Sometimes, even though all the words are there, the slow halting and monotonous style of the speaker still reveals the effects of the brain injury. Although the brain has some capacity for recovery with the passing of time, speech-language therapy can greatly speed up the slow process of recovering speech and language. Most patients with TBI greatly appreciate the efforts of SLPs and recognize how their efforts assisted them in this process.

Aphasia

Another neurologically based disorder used to be called "childhood aphasia" or "dysphasia." Aphasia is a language disturbance associated with an injury to the brain. Aphasia in children is very different from aphasia in adults. This is because, unlike adults, children are still acquiring speech and language. Oftentimes in children, other areas of the brain, either within the same hemisphere or in the other hemisphere, will take over functions originally performed by the damaged region. Because this disorder is so different from adult aphasia, terms such as childhood aphasia or dysphasia have fallen out of favor.

It is not entirely clear if aphasia, specifically Broca's aphasia (see chapter 13), can be separated from *apraxia of speech*, a more basic motor control problem involving an impairment of the execution of learned complex acts. Are they two different clinical entities or is apraxia of speech just one of the more common symptoms of a Broca's aphasia? In Broca's aphasia there is usually also a reduction of sentence elements, known as *agrammatism*. Broca's aphasics tend to reveal evidence of subtle syntactic impairments in formal grammatical tests. Unfortunately, formal testing of syntactic comprehension is not always part of the battery of tests given to patients with suspected apraxia of speech, and one does not find what one does not look for.

Both the Broca's aphasic and the patient with apraxia of speech tend to have slower labored speech. The listener typically gets the distinct impression that the patient is having a difficult time producing intelligible speech. Previously, it was this slow and labored speech, in contrast to the more fluent speech of Wernicke's aphasics, that suggested that their problem in producing speech was in the motor execution. However, studies that have investigated the speech of Broca's aphasics using instrumental techniques to measure subtle aspects of speech such as voice onset time have revealed that their speech is different from that produced by Wernicke's aphasics.

For example, Blumstein and colleagues (Blumstein, Cooper, Goodglass, Statlender, & Gottlieb, 1980) demonstrated that Broca's aphasics had a distinct difficulty in maintaining appropriate voicing categories that are seen in the normal speaker. The English-speaking Broca's aphasics who participated in this study were found to have overlapping VOT productions. In other words, most of their consonant productions had VOTs between typical voiced and voiceless values—an area typically avoided by the normal speaker.

Other studies that have investigated Japanese-speaking patients with apraxia of speech and Thai-speaking Broca's aphasics have found similar results. But a preliminary study of French-speaking Broca's aphasics revealed that they did not have overlapping VOT productions similar to these other studies. Ryalls, Arsenault, and Provost (1995) have suggested that these results might be due to the voicing categories being particularly distinct in French, in comparison to the other languages studied. However, more instrumental studies that provide acoustic measures of aphasic speech are needed in a wider variety of languages in order to know to what degree the consequences of Broca's aphasia are similar or different across various languages. It would be particularly interesting to investigate Spanish-speaking Broca's aphasics because Spanish has similar VOT values to French.

VOT is just one aspect of the production of stop consonants. Shinn and Blumstein (1983) found spectral information for place of articulation to be relatively undisturbed in the speech of Broca's aphasics. These authors suggest that it is those aspects of speech that require fine temporal coordination between various articulators that are particularly affected in Broca's aphasia. A study of vowel formant frequencies, relatively stable acoustic correlates, did not reveal a similar distinction between patients with Broca's aphasia versus those with Wernicke's aphasia (Ryalls, 1986). These results suggest that vowels and consonants may be stored somewhat differently in the brain (Ryalls, 1987), something already suggested by results from dichotic listening experiments.

Another neural site associated with speech production is found in the temporal lobe, which controls audition. Damage to this area is often accompanied by a fluency in speech production but with semantically void language. Remember that such fluent aphasics are also termed Wernicke's aphasics after the German neurologist Carl Wernicke, who first recorded the case of a patient who presented with seemingly normal but meaningless speech and who showed upon death a lesion (damage) in the area of the temporal lobe now known as Wernicke's area.

Function words seem to be intact, such as prepositions, articles, and conjunctions, but many content words, nouns and verbs, are either paraphasias or neologisms. A *paraphasia* is a word close to the target word in either sound or meaning. A sound similarity, such as *elephant* for *elevator*, is termed a *phonological paraphasia*. Semantic replacements, such as *ladder* for *elevator*, are called *semantic paraphasias*. *Neologisms* are nonsense utterances that cannot be explained by substitutions; for example, *kletveld* has no obvious target word (Lezak, 1983).

A third type of aphasia can be characterized as fluent and meaningful, but with an inability to repeat speech the individual can hear and understand. *Conduction aphasia*, as it is termed, often results from damage in an area called the arcuate fasciculus. The arcuate fasciculus is a neural fiber bundle that is thought to connect Broca's and Wernicke's areas of the brain. This is why a problem in the conduction of information from Wernicke's to Broca's areas is known as conduction aphasia. In conduction aphasia, the individual can understand the speech presented to him or her, can speak spontaneously, but cannot repeat the speech.

More recently, the language abilities of the right hemisphere have been investigated. Originally labeled the "nonlanguage" center, the right hemisphere has been shown to function in the processing of prosody, the melodic component of speech, especially that of a nonlinguistic nature.

Other Neurological Disorders

We have spent quite a lot of time here and in chapter 13 discussing aphasia because both of the authors of this book have a special interest in aphasia. We cannot prevent ourselves from attempting to convey our intense interest in this fascinating disorder to our students. However, there are a variety of other neurological disorders affecting speech that we still have not considered here. *Amyotrophic-lateral sclerosis* (ALS or Lou Gehrig's disease) is one very serious neurological disease that is often discovered by the speech disorder it produces. Unfortunately, by the time it has affected speech production, the patient may not survive for more than a few years. *Multiple sclerosis* can also have serious effects on speech production, although not in all cases. *Muscular dystrophy* and *cerebral palsy* can also both have serious consequences on speech production. These are only a few of the neurological disorders that can affect speech production. Speech pathology programs routinely require a separate course in language disorders, so we will limit our discussion of disorders in this text.

Aging and Neurological Disorders

We would, however, like to consider two other neurological disorders that affect so many older persons. *Alzheimer disease* is so common among the elderly that many now consider it to be a normal consequence of the aging process. Although the memory and language symptoms of Alzheimer disease are well known, it is not currently known if the disease also affects speech production. The other neurological disease that unfortunately is commonly found among the elderly is *Parkinson disease*. Since it affects motor activities and respiration, Parkinson disease typically has a noticeable effect on speech production. Unlike those of Alzheimer disease, the language consequences of Parkinson disease are typically much more subtle.

Many Parkinson patients can benefit from the services of a SLP. Some SLPs used to feel that these patients were not good candidates for therapy since their disease was progressive and they did not show much improvement. Ramig and colleagues (Ramig, Bonitati, Lemke, & Horii, 1994) have developed a therapy program specifically for patients with Parkinson disease that they have shown to be effective in improving speech production. They named the program the Lee Silverman Method after one of their patients with Parkinson disease of whom they were particularly fond.

In chapter 18, we will consider in detail the case of a patient with Parkinson disease who demonstrated real improvement in speech due to therapy. In this case, we will show you objective measures that quantify the patient's improvement. We feel that this case is useful as an example of the type of therapy that also provides quantitative data justifying its effectiveness.

We have only touched briefly on some of the disorders that can affect speech production, since this is an introductory course. Although we have only considered a few disorders, we have considered some of those that are more frequently seen in speech-language pathology clinics. Hopefully, as future SLPs you are beginning to understand the tremendous role you can have in improving the lives of people affected with disorders of speech. Next, we consider the use of computer technology in the measurement, diagnosis, and treatment of speech disorders.

Study Questions

1. How does adult-onset aphasia differ from cases of aphasia in childhood?

2. How is Alzheimer disease different from Parkinson disease?

3. Do you think that HMOs (Health Maintenance Organizations) should provide speech therapy for patients with Parkinson disease even though the disease is progressive and may shorten the patient's life? Justify your response as if it were an appeal to an HMO board.

4. How does speech science impact the treatment of production disorders? Discuss in relation to one disorder associated with childhood, one found in adulthood, and one associated with the elderly.

References

Blumstein, S., Cooper, W., Goodglass, H., Statlender, S., & Gottlieb, J. (1980). Production deficits in aphasia: A voice-onset time analysis. *Brain and Language, 9,* 153–170.

Cairns, H. (1996). *The acquisition of language* (2nd ed.). Austin, TX: Pro-Ed.

DeNil, L. (1997). *Functional neuroimaging and stuttering: Theoretical and clinical implications.* Oral presentation to the Department of Communicative Disorders, University of Central Florida, Orlando, FL.

Lezak, M. (1983). *Neuropsychological assessment* (2nd ed.). New York: Oxford University Press.

Nelson, N. (1998). *Childhood language disorders in context* (2nd ed.). Boston: Allyn & Bacon.

Ramig, L., Bonitati, C., Lemke, J., & Horii, Y. (1994). Voice treatment for patients with Parkinson's disease: Development of an approach and preliminary efficacy data. *Journal of Medical Speech-language Pathology, 2,* 191–209.

Ryalls, J. (1986). A study of vowel production in aphasia. *Brain and Language, 29,* 48–67.

Ryalls, J. (1987). Vowel production in aphasia: Towards an account of the consonant-vowel dissociation. In J. Ryalls (Ed.), *Phonetic approaches to speech production in aphasia and related disorders.* Boston: College-Hill Press.

Ryalls, J., Arsenault, N., & Provost, H. (1995). Voice onset time in French-speaking aphasics. *Journal of Communication Disorders, 28(3),* 205–216.

Shinn, P., & Blumstein, S. (1983). Phonetic disintegration in aphasia: Acoustic analysis of spectral characteristics for place of articulation. *Brain and Language, 20,* 90–114.

Wit, J., Maasen, B., Gabreels, F., & Thoonen, G. (1993). Maximum performance tests in children with developmental dysarthria. *Journal of Speech and Hearing Research, 36,* 4452–4459.

17 Computers and Speech Science

The availability of cheaper, smaller, and more powerful computers, coupled with the development of user-friendly computer programs designed specifically for speech analysis, has radically altered speech science over the past two decades.

Historical Notes

While in the 1960s significant speech research was largely limited to a few major research settings in the United States (notably Haskins Laboratories and the Massachusetts Institute of Technology), the 1970s saw a proliferation of speech research related to the development of the microcomputer.

Until that time, most speech research was performed on the Sound Spectrograph. Speech research on the Sound Spectrograph was much more tedious and time-consuming than on the computer because all of the measures had to be interpolated by hand. In other words, time measures had to be converted from inches or centimeters of spectrograph paper to seconds or milliseconds of time. The frequencies of the dark blobs that represented formants on spectrograms had to be estimated by hand. This can be a very tedious process, as anyone who has analyzed speech in this manner knows all too well. There are also the smelly black fumes that are emitted as the spectrographic image is literally "burned" onto the revolving carbon paper on the old spectrographs (or the spectacular result of wrapping the spectrographic paper onto the drum the wrong way—an airborne sheet of burning paper and a menacing electrical arc as the needle sparks the bare metal drum!). The spectrograph, still thought of as "state-of-the-art" until the 1970s, already seems poised to become a relic for the speech science museum and may soon take its place there next to the Rousselot cylinder. These days, there is a more convenient computerized version of the spectrograph, the digital spectrograph.

As speech analysis software became available and microcomputers cheaper and more powerful, speech analysis systems became commonly available in the 1980s. One significant development in this area was the Computer Speech Laboratory or CSL from Kay Elemetrics, the most widely known company in America exclusively devoted to speech analysis. While there is also notable university-developed software, such as CSpeech (University of Wisconsin, Madison), BLISS (Brown University), CESR (University of Western Ontario), the association of Kay Elemetrics with the sound spectrograph assured that CSL attracted the most attention in speech-language pathology. The fact that most personnel in speech-language pathology programs were already familiar with some Kay equipment such as the Visipitch or Spectrograph may have given CSL the advantage of familiarity.

CSL will be considered in more detail below, along with several other computer systems that the SLP is likely to encounter in the modern clinic. This list is by no means representative of the myriad of systems available, but simply those we feel student-clinicians are most likely to encounter. These days, most university departments of speech-language pathology possess equipment that allows for the kind of acoustic manipulations only available in major research settings just a few years ago. Computers that fit on desktops are often more powerful and efficient than computers that used to fill an entire room, just two decades ago. The wide availability of computer systems should ensure that speech science research is within the grasp of at least all graduate students in speech-language pathology in the United States.

Digitization

When we talk about a "computer system" here, we mean a sufficiently powerful microcomputer, outfitted with a specialized board that digitizes speech (sometimes called an A/D analog-to-digital converter) and specialized software for acoustic analyses. It is necessary for a computer to have the continuous analog speech signal digitized or converted into numbers, in order for the computer to be able to analyze speech. However, some systems are now able to accept input directly from digital recordings, preempting the need for a digital conversion. Remember that numbers are essentially the "language" that computers speak.

Hint to Students

In order for computers to treat speech signals, the continuous analog signal must be "digitized" or converted into a numerical equivalent.

Sampling and Sampling Rate

This is the same digitization principle as is used in compact disks—music is encoded onto compact discs as numbers that the CD player's laser scanner "reads" back in order to play the CD. Figure 17.1 below illustrates the digitization process. Most compact disks are digitized or "sampled" at about 44 kHz, which means that a "sample" or number is read from the continuous original signal at 44,000 times per second. This ensures that the digital version is very close to the original, up to frequencies that are one-half of the sampling rate—up to about 22 kHz. This principle is known as *Nyquist's theorem* (Lieberman & Blumstein, 1988).

Speech is typically sampled at a lower rate than music for two reasons. Although a faster sampling rate produces a better quality sample, more computer memory is used. In fact, there is a proportional rate—sampling twice as fast takes up twice as much memory. Second, most of the significant information in speech is contained in frequencies up to about 5000 Hertz. Frequencies above 5000 Hertz make less and less of an impact on speech perception. As a result, most speech research is conducted with a 10,000 Hertz sampling rate. By the Nyquist theorem, this rate ensures that frequency information is preserved accurately up to 5000 Hertz. However, since the significant frequencies in children's speech are higher (due to their smaller vocal folds and shorter vocal tracts), a 20,000 Hertz rate is typically used for children. According to Nyquist's theorem, this ensures accurate acoustic analyses up to 10,000 Hz.

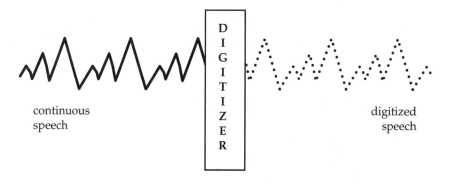

FIGURE 17.1 Schematic drawing of the sampling process wherein a continuous analog signal is converted into discrete numerical points that can be treated by the computer. The sampling rate represents how close the sample points are together.

Quantization Factor

Another factor in digitizing speech, besides the sampling rate, is the *quantization factor*, or the degree of amplitude resolution. This measure is typically expressed in bits. A bit is 2 to the Nth levels of resolution. To take an example, two-bit quantization would give 2 to the 2nd power, or 4 amplitude levels. Four-bit quantization would give $2 \times 2 \times 2 \times 2$, or 16 levels of amplitude. Typically, contemporary speech research uses at least 12-bit quantization, and most systems now use a 16-bit standard.

Fourier Analysis and Linear Predictive Coding

We have already discussed Fourier's algorithm, which is one of the main principles used in speech analysis. A *Fourier analysis* reveals the fundamental frequency and indicates the location of formant frequencies. However, typically an additional mathematical procedure, known as *linear predictive coding* (LPC) is used to indicate the exact frequency location of formants. There are many other mathematical formulas that offer various other kinds of spectral information. But Fourier and LPC are the cornerstones of frequency analysis in contemporary speech research.

Timing and Frequency

The other kind of acoustic information computers can offer speech scientists relates to timing. In fact, all speech research boils down to either frequency measures or timing measures. Typical frequency measures of speech include fundamental frequency (f_o) and the first three formant frequencies (F_1, F_2, F_3). Some typical duration measures include speech rate, vowel duration and voice onset time (VOT). (See chapter 9 for discussion.)

Synthesized Speech and Speech Recognition

While so far we have been considering machine measures of speech, we should also consider speech produced by machine and recognized by machine. These days no one can escape the synthesized voice. While quality synthesized speech formerly required very sophisticated laboratory settings, it can now be found, encoded on electronic chips, on everything from state-of-the-art jet aircraft guidance systems, to talking toys. The drive to use speech probably stems from the fact that there is no more natural or user-friendly way to interface with machines than our own natural language. For this reason, we are most likely to witness increased use of speech as a means to interact with machines on an increasing scale throughout the next millennium.

When people are able to speak to their computers instead of keying in written language, the interaction between human and machine is likely to speed up significantly. Speech is a very rapid means of transmitting complex messages. While many people become very proficient with keyboards, they never can achieve rates as fast as oral speech. That is not only because speech can be presented very rapidly, but because, in most listening situations, speech is understood by the human listener as quickly as it is produced. Remember that speech is highly encoded, with one segment holding perceptual cues for several other segments at the same time. This immediacy was a problem that previously impeded spoken speech recognition by computer. While we have been able to get computers to "talk" for quite some time now, the task of getting them to "understand" speech stumped researchers for several decades.

It was only when researchers were able to simulate speech perception that speech science entered the modern era. It was Haskins Laboratories' pioneering work attempting to isolate the relevant acoustic correlates of speech that revealed just how unique speech is as an acoustic code (Liberman, Cooper, Shankweiler, & Studdert-Kennedy, 1967) and demonstrated just how difficult a task automated speech perception would be.

It is not too difficult to imagine just how much faster we might be able to interact with computers if we were able to lay aside our keyboards and simply "converse" with them. Changing the somewhat artificial interaction via keyboard to something as natural as speech is likely to fundamentally alter the manner in which we interact with computers. Science fiction movies enjoy warning us about the potential danger of gaining, and then relying too heavily upon, such an intimate communication with our machines. One only has to remember the deceptively soothing voice of the devious HAL computer in the film *2001: A Space Odyssey* for a perfect example.

In any case, the increasing speech-based interaction between human and machine has a special implication for SLPs. While persons with certain motor disabilities are likely to benefit significantly from not being dependent on the fine motor skills that keyboard entry requires, how are we going to ensure that those individuals with speech disorders are going to have the same access to computers when a spoken interface becomes the norm? Obviously, many of these individuals are not going to be able to "speak for themselves" and it should be the responsibility of their SLPs to represent their interests. We should ensure that individuals with difficult-to-recognize speech are not left by the wayside.

This area is advancing so quickly that it is probably already time to advocate that speech recognition technology also include the slower, sometimes somewhat slurred speech of persons with various dysarthrias, for example. It is likely that individuals whose motor impairments also affect speech production would be among those who can benefit most greatly from the assistance of computers to assist in controlling their environment. Although currently a good deal of the effort for spoken computer interaction includes these individuals, the situation may change when spoken computer recognition speeds up considerably.

The Role of the SLP in Relation to Technology

Speech-language pathologists also have a role in evaluating the efficiency of various technologies developed to assist them in providing speech therapy. While it takes engineers and computer specialists to develop these systems, it is only the experienced SLP who can determine the effectiveness of computerized speech training. Herein lies the increasing importance of speech science within the profession of speech-language pathology.

Speech-language pathologists are likely to witness an even greater role of speech science within the profession, as they are called upon to demonstrate the effectiveness of the therapy that they provide. Speech science can provide objective measures that demonstrate the effectiveness of therapy. With the type of carefully managed health care that is prevalent in the United States, it may become increasingly necessary for SLPs to be able to provide numbers that substantiate the benefit of speech therapy to clients.

In the next chapter, the role of the SLP will be illustrated through a case study. In this study, a computer was used (1) to assist in providing speech therapy,

(2) in obtaining objective measures that guided therapy, and (3) to demonstrate the effectiveness of the therapy. We will consider this case in detail because we feel that this increasing interaction with computers is likely to characterize the way speech-language pathology will evolve as the profession now enters the twenty-first century.

Some SLPs may be resistant to this type of change. Some may harbor unfounded fears that computers get too much attention within the profession. But thus far, studies that have investigated computer-assisted therapy have only served to underscore the crucial contribution of the SLP. Computers are a tool, but one that must be manipulated by the well-trained SLP in order to be effective. In fact, some researchers have pointed out the potential negative consequences of computer-based therapy that is not under the vigilant supervision of the SLP (i.e., Ryalls, Michallet, & Le Dorze, 1994). This should serve as a warning to those who think that speech therapy can be handed over to computers, or to individuals with less sophisticated training, such as speech-language assistants. In the next section, we consider a few of the computer systems that the SLP might encounter in the clinic.

Computer Systems in the Clinic

Kay Elemetrics Visipitch

The Visipitch used to be the instrument most likely to be seen in the clinical setting. In the earliest versions, the Visipitch was not much more than a CRT (cathode-ray tube) oscilloscope with a microphone. A client or clinician spoke into the microphone and a line appeared on the CRT screen. A cursor could then be adjusted to line up with the majority of fundamental frequency points to estimate an average fundamental frequency of phonation.

However, there were some shortcomings associated with Visipitch. For one thing, once a sentence was recorded it had to be erased before a new sentence could be recorded. Thus, it was impossible to store data from repeated sentences or reveal the longitudinal effects of therapy. Another disadvantage was that Visipitch often had difficulty distinguishing noise from speech, and thus produced erroneous points that did not actually relate to the fundamental frequency. The early Visipitch was also rather susceptible to harmonic errors.

Many of these disadvantages were overcome with the computer interface for Visipitch. For example, it is now possible to record data points from many sentences and to redisplay data points from computer memory for purposes of comparison. Although many of the disadvantages have been overcome, Visipitch has not kept pace with other speech analysis systems. The most serious shortcoming of Visipitch is that it is only useful for measures of fundamental frequency; it is not very accurate for duration measures. For example, it is not possible to measure voice onset time from a Visipitch. And the Visipitch does not allow the user to derive other important speech measures—most importantly, it is not possible to measure formant frequencies on a Visipitch. Of course, students should also bear in mind that Visipitch was not intended to perform these speech measures. Figure 17.2 below illustrates the Visipitch with computer interface being used by a SLP with a young client.

IBM SpeechViewer

In some ways, SpeechViewer can be seen as picking up where Visipitch left off. Besides allowing the user to see the ongoing fundamental frequency and duration of speech, there are interactive "games" that allow a client to work on various aspects of speech production. This should only take place under the watchful supervision of a trained SLP. For example, one of us discovered that children can easily misuse a SpeechViewer. One of the modules in SpeechViewer designed to display amplitude is an expanding red balloon. While it was true that the bright red expanding balloon on the computer screen did capture the interest of the hearing-impaired children receiving therapy, some of these children immediately attempted to scream into the microphone loud enough to burst the balloon. This

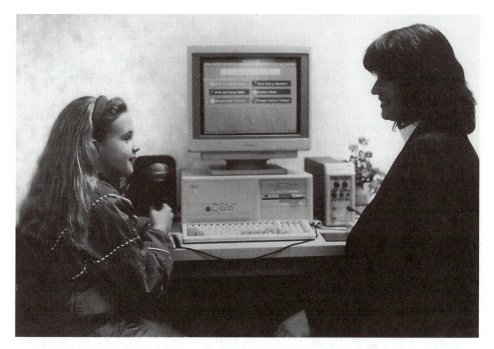

FIGURE 17.2   A speech-language pathologist working with a client (holding the microphone) on the Kay Elemetrics computerized Visipitch system. (Courtesy of Kay Elemetrics Corporation)

was obviously not one of the exercises intended by its developers! Such loud speech production could eventually lead to vocal abuse. This is one simple example of why computer systems for training speech production should only be used under the guidance of a trained SLP. (In fact, it is IBM's policy only to sell SpeechViewer to licensed SLPs and not to highly motivated parents with good intentions. This is a policy that we applaud.)

SpeechViewer has already undergone three different overhauls since it was introduced onto the market in the late 1980s. At present, the SpeechViewer III has overcome some of the limitations of the earliest version so that now users are able to chain together speech elements into whole words.

While it is a significant clinical tool, there are limitations to the use of Speech-Viewer in speech research. Although a number of useful measures such as fundamental frequency and duration can be derived in a user-friendly manner, it is our experience that it is not possible to perform accurate voice onset time measures, nor to derive accurate formant frequency measures for connected speech on this machine. However, SpeechViewer does offer a powerful clinical tool that provides many measures useful to much clinical practice. The latest versions allow clinicians to tract progress of a client and thus provide objective measures that document the effectiveness of speech therapy.

Kay Elemetrics CSL

While the Computer Speech Lab or CSL may be beyond the reach of many clinical settings, it is becoming fairly common in the university laboratory. CSL has quickly become the most widely used speech analysis system in the United States. While there are advantages to some of the university-developed systems over CSL, this system probably offers the widest range of potential uses. There are programs for all of the standard speech measures, as well as some more "experimental" measures used in the assessment of voice quality (such as jitter, shimmer, and harmonics-to-noise ratio) in the Multiple Dimensional Voice Profile or MDVP section. A CSL can also be interfaced with the Nasometer to provide measures of nasalence, as well as with the Kay Elemetrics electroglottograph (EGG), electropalatograph (EPG), and pneumotachograph. Figure 17.3 illustrates a CSL system.

Another advantage of CSL is that the programs that are available are fairly well documented and debugged and there is extensive user-support. One limitation of CSL is that improvements and additional theoretical analyses are likely to show up more slowly on the CSL than on university-developed systems. User manuals might not be available for all aspects of university-based systems, but it is university-based systems that push speech research to new limits. The cutting edge of research will always require computer systems to perform more and more sophisticated analyses and employ mathematical techniques.

We can only speculate on the computer systems that will become available to SLPs in the next millennium. It is probable that the use of parallel programming and expert systems will automate many of the most time-consuming aspects of speech research, which will make it possible to perform analyses on much larger data sets than is currently possible. At present, many people think that speech research is not very labor-intensive because it is performed on computer. The naive public may think that all the speech scientist has to do is place the recording onto the computer and all of the measures are then performed automatically! But the truth of the matter is that students are sometimes shocked when they discover that many acoustic measures such as voice onset time are still largely performed by hand and ear. Even in the laboratory, the computer is a tool that is only as sophisticated as its user. This is not to deny that the computer is a tremendously useful and powerful tool, but ultimately, it is still the human ear and brain at the base of speech science research. Perhaps it is reassuring that speech research still retains this human element in the face of ever-increasing prevalence of computers as we begin the new millennium.

Table 17.1 presents a summary of functions and disadvantages of these three technologies.

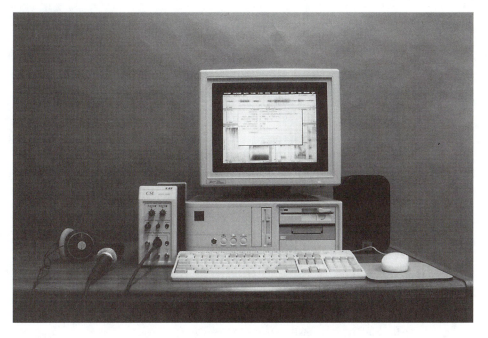

FIGURE 17.3 Kay Elemetrics Computer Speech System or CSL. (Courtesy of Kay Elemetrics Corporation)

TABLE 17.1   Some Speech Science Technologies for SLPs

Name	Functions	Disadvantages
Kay Elemetrics Visipitch	Records data points from many sentences Measures f_o Redisplays points from memory for comparison	Only measures f_o Cannot measure formants or VOT
IBM Speech Viewer III	Displays f_o & duration immediately Contains interactive "video" games Tracks progress	Cannot measure formants (of connected speech) Cannot measure VOT
Kay Elemetrics Computer Speech Lab (CSL)	Provides all standard speech measures Assesses voice quality Interfaces to other instruments	Not all state-of-the-art speech measures DOS programs LPC does not print formant values

Study Questions

1. Name one of the ways that speech-language pathologists should be involved in the use of computers within the profession.

2. What are some of the advantages of supplementing traditional speech-language therapy with a computer?

3. Why should SLPs closely supervise and monitor the use of computers for speech therapy?

4. Is speech-language therapy ever likely to become completely computerized? Why or why not?

References

Liberman, A., Cooper, F., Shankweiler, D., & Studdert-Kennedy, M. (1967). Perception of the speech code. *Psychological Review, 74*, 431–461.

Lieberman, P., & Blumstein, S. (1988). *Speech physiology, speech perception, and acoustic phonetics.* London, UK: Cambridge University Press.

Ryalls, J., Michallet, B., & Le Dorze, G. (1994). A preliminary evaluation of the clinical effectiveness of vowel training for hearing-impaired children on IBM's SpeechViewer. *Volta Review, 96*(1), 19–30.

CHAPTER
18 The Role of the Speech-Language Pathologist

The SLP has an important role in society because effective communication is so central to human beings. Partly a teacher, partly a nurse, both counselor and coach, the SLP may be a patient's bridge back to social interaction. In this chapter we want to consider some research demonstrating the effectiveness of speech-language therapy. At the same time, we hope to suggest a model for modern speech therapy—one in which the clinician obtains objective measures on the effectiveness of therapy at the same time that it is being administered. In this manner, we hope to show once again why it is that students of speech-language pathology and audiology need to have a good understanding of speech science.

The SLP as a Member of the Medical Team

The role of the SLP is changing as society changes. Recently, SLPs have taken an increasing role on the medical team. There are situations where the SLP may even be called upon to intervene between patient and physician. Two examples come to mind. The first is in the case of dysphagia, where the SLP may be more conversant with supralaryngeal anatomy as it functions in the coordinated act of swallowing than is the physician. It is typically the SLP who requests a fluoroscopic examination (often referred to as a modified barium test) in order to test for the possible presence of undetected (i.e., silent) aspiration. Aspiration of food and liquids into the lungs can be dangerous indeed. Liquids entering the lungs can provoke pneumonia, and even more alarming, there is also the potential for choking to death.

Sometimes physicians are reluctant to acknowledge that some abnormality has escaped their careful scrutiny—especially in the absence of outwardly visible signs. It is a rather interesting development that dysphagia has been relegated to the SLP. However, there does not currently appear to be a health professional better trained to deal with the problems of deglutition and swallowing. This development raises interesting questions about the relationship between eating and speaking. Certainly, eating is a more basic function than is speech. But since they share anatomical structures, the question of whether speech is a function "overlaid"

147

on chewing and swallowing, or whether there are entirely new and independent systems involved in speech, invites further investigation. Detailed investigation of speech production in patients with dysphagia may provide us with some clues as to its relationship to speech. A preliminary study of speech in five patients with dysphagia revealed subtle VOT production abnormalities (Ryalls, Gustafson, & Santini, 1999).

The other area where the SLP may intercede between patient and physician is in the case of ventilator-dependent patients. These are patients who are dependent upon ventilator machines for respiration and cannot breathe on their own. Some ventilator tubes have an inflatable cuff that helps to maintain the tube's placement within the trachea. However, this cuff also prevents air from passing up through the vocal folds to provide a sound source for speech. Of course, this absent sound source cannot then be filtered by the vocal tract and shaped into the sounds of speech. While it may be reassuring to know that the ventilator tube will be maintained in a proper position, some physicians may ignore, or down play, the tremendous isolating effects of not being able to produce speech. Many patients find this inability to produce speech, which they may be experiencing for the first time in their entire lives, very frightening. In this case, it may be the SLP who acts as the patients' advocate and spokesperson, once the patients' progress warrants, in order to have the cuff deflated so that the patients can speak again. In this example, we are once again reminded of the intimate relationship between speech and respiration.

Case Study—Parkinson Disease

Let us consider a case study (Le Dorze, Dionne, Ryalls, Julien & Ouellet, 1992) of an older woman with Parkinson disease. This case study demonstrates how speech measures were used to guide therapy. (Another study that shows how measures can be used to guide therapy for voice disorders is found in Behrman & Orlikoff, 1997.) Parkinson disease is a neurological disorder whose primary clinical traits include increased muscle rigidity, a notable tremor, and difficulty in initiating movements or stopping them (Pincus & Tucker, 1985). Such motor difficulties may manifest themselves in speech deficits. The patient of this study was not satisfied with the results of her traditional speech-language therapy and sought out further assistance in regaining more normal speech production, especially in terms of the prosodic qualities of her speech. The study we will discuss is a multiple-baseline design in which three different speech behaviors were constantly assessed and monitored while each of them was treated individually in a systematic manner. In order to understand the study, Figure 18.1 is provided and will be discussed further.

Three different aspects of the patient's speech prosody were targeted for therapy: (1) *intonation*, (2) *average fundamental frequency*, and (3) *rate*. These aspects were chosen because they were all noted to be abnormal in the patient's speech, and they could easily be objectively measured by available instrumentation—in this case, an IBM SpeechViewer I.

Objective measures were defined for each of these speech aspects. For intonation, the amount of difference in fundamental frequency between a declarative and interrogative version of the same sentence was determined. In the so-called yes-no or rhetorical questions used in this study, the only difference between the two types of sentences is the rather sharply rising fundamental frequency contour in the question version. For example, "It's nice out today," spoken with a falling fundamental frequency, is a statement. But when the same words are spoken with a rising fundamental frequency, the statement becomes the question: "It's nice out today?" Sometimes these questions are used to express irony or disbelief on the part of the speaker. In any case, the average amount of difference in fundamental frequency between question and statement versions was measured on the last syllable of the sentence. This measure was taken to reflect a speaker's ability to appropriately modulate fundamental frequency. Averages used to plot the figure were based on 10 pairs of sentences.

The speaker's average fundamental frequency over the length of the 5 to 7 syllable sentences was measured. This measure is directly available from the fundamental frequency patterning module of SpeechViewer I. Both the SLP and the patient agreed that her fundamental frequency was inappropriately low for the patient's gender and age. Therapy targeted a higher average fundamental frequency.

Speech rate was calculated by dividing the total sentence duration by the total number of syllables in the sentence production. This results in a rate measure expressed in terms of syllables per second. Speech rate can also be measured with a simple stopwatch, although a measure by computer may be somewhat more accurate. (Some normal ranges of speech rate can be found in Kent, 1994.) The patient's abnormally fast speaking rate contributed to listeners' difficulty in understanding her speech. Thus, therapy was directed towards reducing the patient's habitual rate of speech.

In the baseline period of the experiment, average measures were taken before therapy began. The first stage of therapy, Phase A of Figure 18.1, begun after four sessions of baseline measures, was directed at improving intonation. Remember that intonation was defined as the average difference in fundamental frequency between question and statement versions. The clinician provided spoken models with a large intonation difference and pointed out where there should be a larger fundamental frequency difference on the computer screen. The patient viewed her own fundamental frequency contours. In other words, the patient was provided simple biofeedback on the computer screen based on her own fundamental frequency production.

One standard deviation of improvement maintained for three continuous sessions was the target goal selected for each stage of therapy. Notice that baseline measures were continuously provided for average fundamental frequency and rate, even though no therapy for them is being provided during the intonation phase of therapy. f_0 therapy began in session 17, and rate therapy began in session 23.

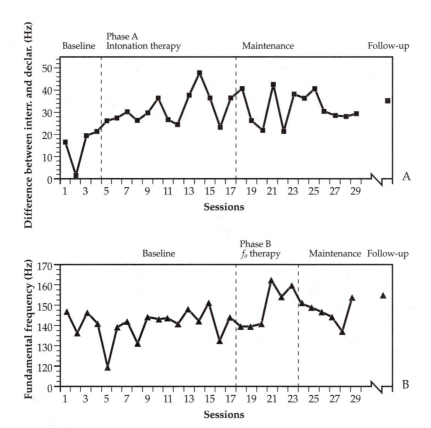

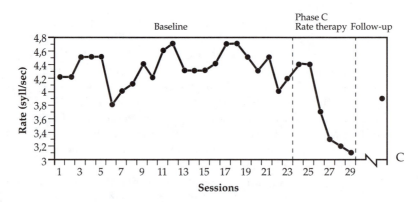

FIGURE 18.1 Multiple baseline study of therapy for (A) intonation, (B) fundamental frequency, and (C) rate in a female patient with Parkinson disease. See text for details. (Reprinted from Le Dorze, Dionne, Ryalls, Julien, & Ouellet, 1992, with the permission of Taylor & Francis Ltd., London, UK)

The patient makes modest but continued improvement in intonation until session 11, when there is a drop-off in performance. After session 12, however, a larger increase is seen, only to drop off again in the next two therapy sessions. In other words, there is a fair degree of variability in the patient's performance in the second half of the intonation therapy. However, the patient has maintained the criterion of one standard deviation of intonation improvement for three sessions by session 17, when the second phase of therapy was initiated.

In the second phase of therapy, Phase B of Figure 18.1, the SLP provided spoken models of higher fundamental frequency and directed the patient's attention to the fundamental frequency measure on the computer screen. There was a rather dramatic improvement in average fundamental frequency in the fourth session of fundamental frequency therapy (session 21). The patient maintained an almost equally higher average fundamental frequency for the next two sessions, and so the third phase of therapy was begun.

The third, and final, stage of therapy was directed at slowing down the patient's speech rate. This stage is Phase C in Figure 18.1. The SLP provided spoken models at a slower speech rate and directed the patient's attention to the duration measure on the computer screen. The patient was able to achieve a much slower average rate of speech production by the third session of therapy (session 26). An improvement of one standard deviation was achieved and maintained for three sessions, so therapy was terminated at session 29.

Hint to Students

In the treatment of this Parkinson patient, the SLP utilized a computer system to provide models and feedback on speech production. The feedback was both auditory and visual and seems to assist the patient in gaining more control over her speech production.

Each of these aspects was measured again at 10 weeks following the final stage of therapy to determine how well the effects of therapy were maintained. Each of the follow-up measures showed improvement compared to pretherapy baseline measures. These positive results are rather significant because patients with Parkinson disease are often not thought to be good candidates for speech-language therapy. Some SLPs may feel that it is not ethical to provide therapy for patients with a degenerative disease like Parkinson. However, this study shows that a motivated patient can measurably improve speech production under the careful guidance of an experienced SLP using modern technology.

This study also provides a model for students. Many patients' speech therapy is paid by managed health care systems that are increasingly requiring objective evidence of improvement resulting from therapy. Thus, these types of objective measures are likely to become more and more important in the clinical arena throughout the next millennium. The next decade will probably see increasing computerization of the speech-language clinic, as computer systems appropriate for assisting therapy, and for measuring the effects of therapy, become cheaper, more user-friendly, and more widely available.

It is important that SLPs implicate themselves in the development process of these systems. While engineers and computer experts are needed to develop such computer systems, only practicing SLPs can determine how appropriate and effective they are. It is also incumbent upon the SLP to develop and test the effectiveness of speech therapy regimens that target specific areas for speech improvement. Your generation of SLPs will have to be part practitioners, but also part researchers. It is this role as researchers that underscores one more reason that students need a solid basis in speech science.

This text has served to initiate undergraduates to the fundamentals of speech science. If you have read this book carefully and been successful in this course, you now possess a solid basis for furthering your knowledge in this area in a graduate course in speech science.

Study Questions

1. How is the field of speech-language pathology becoming increasingly medical? Describe a specific example.

2. You are asked by a Health Maintenance Organization (HMO) to demonstrate the effectiveness of your patient's speech-language therapy. Describe how you might convince the HMO to continue paying for your client's therapy.

3. Discuss the use of computer technology in the treatment of Parkinson disease by a speech-language pathologist. Which is more important in the therapy, the SLP or the computer?

4. In the study described in this chapter, follow-up measures were provided 10 weeks after therapy was completed. Why do you think it is important to provide such follow-up measures? Could the therapy still be considered successful if the follow-up measures were at baseline levels?

References

Behrman, A., & Orlikoff, R. (1997). Instrumentation in voice assessment and treatment: What's the use? *American Journal of Speech-Language Pathology, 6*, 9–16.

Kent, R. (1994). *Reference manual for communicative sciences and disorders.* Austin, TX: Pro-Ed.

Le Dorze, G., Dionne, L., Ryalls, J., Julien, M., & Ouellet, L. (1992). The effects of speech and language therapy for a case of dysarthria associated with Parkinson's disease. *European Journal of Disorders of Communication, 27*, 313–324.

Pincus, J., & Tucker, G. (1985). *Behavioral neurology* (3rd ed.). New York: Oxford University Press.

Ryalls, J., Gustafson, K., & Santini, C. (1999). A preliminary investigation of voice onset time production in persons with dysphagia. *Dysphagia.*

GLOSSARY

allophone   surface form of a phoneme; [æ] and [æ̃] are allophones of the phoneme /æ/.

abduction   the action of opening, separating. Abducted vocal folds are parted.

absolute universals   language characteristics found in all human languages; examples include having consonant/vowel distinctions and noun/verb distinctions.

acoustic invariance   one-to-one correspondence between acoustic characteristic and perception of sound. Much acoustic research is currently focused on the search for invariance.

adduction   action of closing, approximating. Adducted vocal folds are pulled together.

affricate   manner of articulation that involves a stop-consonant onset and fricative offset.

agrammatism   inability to produce or comprehend grammatical information.

alveolar ridge   bony ridge behind teeth in vocal tract; a place of articulation for consonants.

amplitude   amount of displacement of a particle from rest; perceived as loudness; typically measured in decibels (dB).

anomia   inability to name objects due to brain injury.

aperiodic   irregular patterning; fricatives, affricates, and stops are aperiodic.

aphasia   loss of language ability due to brain injury.

arcuate fasciculus   neural fiber tract believed to convey information from Wernicke's area to Broca's area.

articulation   movement of articulators to produce speech sounds.

articulators   parts of vocal tract used to produce speech sounds.

arytenoid cartilage   two triangular-shaped cartilages making up part of the laryngeal structure; one attachment site for the vocal folds and related muscles.

aspiration   breathy quality to production of voiceless stop consonants.

auditory feedback   an individual's speech, presented back to the speaker either in natural conditions or as delayed or altered stimuli.

babbling stage   stage of first language development, roughly 6–12 months, in which infants practice consonant and vowel productions, prior to production of first word.

basilar membrane   part of cochlea that reacts to different frequencies of speech sounds. Its hair cells transduce mechanical impulses of ear to electrical impulses sent to the brain.

Bernoulli force   physical condition in which a rapidly moving air stream passing through a narrow passage results in a drop in air pressure; objects on either side of passage are pulled closer together; comes into play in phonation, helping vocal folds to pull together during vibration.

binary   + and − system of opposites used in phonetic feature description of speech sounds.

Boyle's Law   property of physics that volume and pressure are inversely related. Comes into play with physical condition whereby air molecules tend to move from areas of high pressure to areas of low pressure; comes into play during inhalation and exhalation of respiration.

breath-group view of intonation   theory of sentence intonation in which it is believed that sentences are uttered in a single breath. f_o remains relatively constant until the terminal portion of the sentence, at which point there is a fall-off in f_o for all sentences except yes-no interrogatives.

Broca's aphasia   language impairment characterized by effortful production and agrammatic processing of language; associated with damage to Broca's area, in the left frontal lobe.

categorical perception   way of perceiving speech sounds in which irrelevant differences are ignored.

CAT scan   computerized axial tomography, X-ray imaging technique used to observe brain structures.

cerebral vascular accident (CVA)   stroke; damage to blood vessel in brain. Some feel should be called a "brain attack," analogous to "heart attack."

cinematography   procedure using high-speed film to observe vocal fold vibration.

cingulate cortex   area of primate brain associated with vocalization.

coarticulation   execution of articulatory maneuvers for two separate segments simultaneously.

cochlea   spiral-shaped structure of the inner ear where the process of hearing takes place and frequency information is relayed to the brain.

cochlear implant   sensory aid implanted in the cochlea that attempts to reproduce its tonal organization. Replaces the auditory stimulation that is missing due to improper functioning of sensory cells in cochlea.

complex tone   sound comprising several frequency components; all speech sounds are complex.

consonant   speech sound produced with some amount of constriction in vocal tract; vocal tract is a sound source as well as a filter for sound.

conventionality principle   learning strategy in first language development whereby child prefers the more conventional label to be associated with an item.

corpus callosum   fiber bundle connecting two hemispheres of the brain.

cricoid cartilage   ring-shaped cartilage comprising one section of laryngeal structure; attachment point for various muscles.

cricothyroid muscle   tensing muscle for vocal folds.

critical period   period of first language development after which the ability to acquire a language system natively is severely curtailed; usually placed in human development at around puberty.

cumulative complexity   process of first language development by which child adds to utterances and hence adds complexity to his or her speech.

damping   loss of amplitude.

declination view of intonation   theory of sentence intonation that describes the pattern of f_0 across an utterance as steadily falling off in frequency.

diacritic   symbol on IPA character signaling a specific production of the speech sound. An example is the tilde (~) representing nasalization.

dichotic listening   the simultaneous presentation of separate auditory stimuli to each ear; method of experimentation used to investigate specialized functioning of right and left hemispheres of the brain.

digitization   the process of converting a continuous analog signal into discrete numbers that can then be treated by computer.

distinctive feature   phonetic feature that, when altered, can change the meaning of a word in which it occurs; for English, nasality is distinctive for consonants and nondistinctive for vowels.

diphthong   manner of articulation in which two vowels are produced in succession; acoustic correlate is seen as gradual formant transitions.

duration   physical measure of a speech sound; perceived as length.

dysphagia   swallowing disorder.

dysprosody   disturbance in producing or comprehending prosody of speech, either propositional or emotional.

electroglottograpy (EGG)   one type of recording specific to laryngeal measures; measures rate of vocal fold vibration.

elastic recoil   property of matter to return to resting position.

electromyography (EMG)   a procedure in which electrodes are affixed to patient's skin, or inserted into muscle, to measure muscle activity.

electropalatography (EPG)   a procedure in which a plate with sensing electrodes is used to measure contact of the tongue with the hard and soft palate.

encoded speech   property of speech where phonetic features of neighboring segments overlap.

endoscopic evaluation   procedure using fiberoptic scope to examine patient's vocal folds.

epenthesis   addition of a speech sound; part of the phonological processes found in first language development.

esophagus   pipe to stomach, lying behind trachea.

extendibility principle   learning strategy in first language development whereby child can extend meaning of a word to other objects; may result in overextension of meaning.

filter constraints   limitations placed on language structures due to physiology.

fissure   a furrow or "valley" on the surface of the brain. Also called a sulcus. Fissures are the depressions in the brain, while the mounds or "hills" are its gyri.

formant frequency (formant)   frequency component amplified by resonator (vocal tract). Acoustic properties that distinguish speech sounds. Maxima of harmonic energy. Although revealed by a Fourier analysis, typically measured by LPC or spectrographic analysis.

formant transition   change in frequency value of formant over time; reflects change in position of articulators.

formative universal   language universal referring to rules that order elements of the language.

frequency   number of repetitions by time unit.

fricative   manner of articulation reflected by turbulence in the vocal tract; articulators form narrow passage through which airstream moves.

frontal lobe   part of cerebral cortex associated with motor activity; implicated in control of grammar; site of Broca's area.

fundamental frequency   number of cycles of vocal fold vibration in one second.

glide (semivowel)   manner of articulation characterized by minimal obstruction in the vocal folds; characterized acoustically by gradual formant transitions.

glottis   opening between vocal folds.

gyrus   a mound or hill on the brain's surface. The opposite of a fissure or sulcus, which is a depression in the brain's surface.

harmonics   product of vocal folds; fundamental frequency and multiples.

hearing   process of converting sound energy into a frequency-encoded signal to the brain's auditory cortex.

Hertz   unit of frequency; also *cycles per second*.

holophrastic stage   stage of first language development in which one word conveys full meaning of utterance; nouns usually are more common than verbs; free morphemes more common that bound morphemes.

implicational universal   language trait present in a language if another element is present; for example, a language will have indirect objects only if it has direct objects.

interarytenoid muscle   primary adduction muscle of vocal folds.

intercostal muscles   muscles between ribs; used in respiration to raise and lower rib cage.

International Phonetic Alphabet (IPA)   alphabet used to designate speech sounds in phonetics; one symbol represents one and only one speech sound, in an invariant relationship.

intonation   prosody component of speech; fluctuation of fundamental frequency across the sentence domain.

intraoral pressure   air pressure within oral cavity (mouth).

language universal   language trait seen in abundance throughout human language.

larynx   part of vocal anatomy composed of three cartilages, the vocal folds, and a series of muscles that adduct, abduct, and tense the vocal folds.

lateral   means side; a phonetic feature describing a sound produced with the sides of the tongue lowered; distinguishes [l] from [r].

lateral cricoarytenoid muscle   adduction muscle of vocal folds.

lax   phonetic feature reflecting state of relaxed tongue muscles during production of a vowel.

limbic system   area of the brain considered older than the cerebral cortex; found in other species besides humans.

linear predictive coding (LPC)   mathematical algorithm that determines precise formant frequency values.

linguistic determinism (Sapir-Whorf Hypothesis)   theory that states that the form of one's language determines one's cognitive processes.

linguistic relativism   weaker version of linguistic determinism; states that the form of one's language might influence certain thought processes.

liquid   manner of articulation; speech sound produced with minimal vocal tract obstruction.

manner of articulation   one classification of consonants in phonetics; reflects how speech sounds are produced; reflects amount of obstruction in vocal tract and use of various vocal tract cavities.

mean length of utterance (MLU)   measurement of utterance length used to examine child language in the telegraphic stage of development.

mentalese   hypothesized language in which humans think.

microbeam X-ray   procedure using radio-sensitive particles to track articulation.

minimal pair   set of words that differs in one way phonetically and alternates meaning due to that difference; used to test relationship of phones to phonemes.

modularity   theory that linguistic and cognitive capabilities form independent modules in the human brain.

morphology   study of the construction of words in a language.

magnetic resonance imaging (MRI)   A nonradiation method of body imaging that detects displacements in the orbit of electrons under the influence of a strong magnetic field.

muscular process   section of the arytenoid cartilage that is the attachment point for several muscles involved in phonation.

mutual exclusivity principle   learning strategy that guides first language development; states that child assumes there will be one label for one object in the world.

myoelastic aerodynamic theory of phonation   description of vocal fold vibration, involving muscles, elastic recoil, air pressure, and the Bernoulli effect.

nasal cavity   part of the vocal tract; air-filled space in the nasal and sinus passages.

nasal consonant   manner of articulation characterized by open nasal cavity and fully obstructed oral cavity.

neocortex   area of brain unique to humans; associated with language and higher learning and thinking.

neologism   nonsense word; observed in the speech of Wernicke's aphasics.

neurolinguistics   field of study examining the relationship between language processing and neurology.

occipital lobe   area of brain associated with vision.

operating principles   strategies the child possesses to guide first language development, especially the learning of word meanings.

oral cavity   part of the vocal tract; air-filled cavity formed by the mouth; size and shape of oral cavity associated with the value of second formant.

obstruency   measure of the degree of vocal tract constriction.

ossicles   smallest bones in the human body, found in the middle ear: malleus, incus, and stapes.

overgeneralization (overextension)   process in semantic development of first language whereby the child applies the meaning of a word too broadly to other objects; example: *dog* used for dogs, cows, and horses.

Parkinson disease   a movement disorder associated with damage to the substantia nigra in the brain.

palate   roof of the mouth; place of articulation in the oral cavity of the vocal tract.

paraphasia (phonological and semantic)   a word off target; either phonologically related to the target word (*elevator* for *envelope*) or semantically related (*telegram* for *envelope*).

parietal lobe   area of the brain associated with the integration of sensory information.

periodic   repeating in a regular fashion; a subset of speech sounds are periodic: vowels, nasals, glides, and liquids.

PET Scan   positron emission tomography; a procedure for imaging active areas of the brain.

pharyngeal cavity   back cavity of the vocal tract; volume of pharyngeal cavity is associated with the value of the first formant.

phonation   vibration of the vocal folds.

phone   any spoken speech sound; represented at the phonetic level.

phonetic level   surface level of speech; level of phones, represented with IPA symbols in square brackets.

phonemic level   underlying level of speech; level of phonemes, represented with IPA symbols in slash marks.

phonetic feature   characteristic of a speech sound, usually reflecting articulation.

phonetics   study of speech sounds.

phonology   study of the patterns of speech sounds in language.

pitch   psychological correlate to frequency.

place of articulation   classification of consonants by point of articulatory contact in the vocal tract.

posterior cricoarytenoid muscle   abduction muscle of the vocal folds.

preference constraints   limitations placed on languages reflecting human preferences for certain ordering and other characteristics of language.

prelingual stage   stage of first language development prior to emergence of consonants and vowels; usually placed at 0–6 months of age.

Principles and Parameters Theory   theory of Noam Chomsky that first language acquisition is guided by universals (principles) that vary along language-specific dimensions (parameters).

prosody fluctuation of amplitude, duration, and frequency of speech signal to convey propositional or emotional information; also called the suprasegementals of speech.

protoword pseudoword observed in the late babbling stage of first language development.

psycholinguistics study of language processing.

pure tone sound with one regularly repeating frequency component. Speech is not composed of pure tones but rather of complex tones.

reduplication repetition of a syllable; phonological process seen in first language development.

resonance vibration of a body of air caused by a sound source; in speech the vocal tract is an acoustic resonator that modifies the harmonics of the vocal fold, the source of sound.

respiration inhalation and exhalation of air for quiet breathing and for speech production.

retroflex phonetic feature corresponding to a backward-positioned tongue tip; in English, [r] is considered a retroflexed sound.

rhetorical questions sentences with declarative word order but rising intonation to signal an interrogative.

Rolandic fissure (central sulcus) A primary anatomical landmark of the brain; a furrow that runs vertically and divides the frontal lobe from the parietal lobe.

rounding phonetic feature corresponding to the pursing of the lips during production.

segmental consonant and vowel level of language.

sound symbolism (phonetic symbolism) theory describing a relationship between phonetic categories and semantic meaning; example: [sl] cluster associated with wetness.

source-filter theory theory of speech production denoting the vocal folds as one source of sound and the vocal tract as the filter, modifier of that sound source.

spectrum visual image of speech measuring amplitude by frequency.

spectrograph machine that produces spectrograms.

spectrogram visual image of speech measuring frequency by time; amplitude is noted in the shading of the spectrogram.

statistical universal language characteristic found in a majority of the world's languages.

steady state formant acoustic characteristic of vowels, seen on spectrograms as unchanging (horizontal) formants across the full segment.

stop consonant manner of articulation characterized by full constriction in the vocal tract, then sudden release of air.

stress prosodic component conveyed by the combination of amplitude, duration, and frequency fluctuations; can convey information about word meaning, sentence emphasis, or emotional state of speaker.

stroboscopy procedure using a strobe light and photographs to capture in slow-motion the vibrations of the vocal folds.

subglottal below the glottis (vocal folds).

substantive universal   element found again and again in the world's languages.

substitution   phonological process whereby one sound is produced in place of another; in first language development, children will often substitute a glide for a liquid (*wabbit* for *rabbit*).

supraglottal   above the glottis (vocal folds). See also *supralaryngeal.*

supralaryngeal   structures above the vocal folds, usually called the vocal tract.

suprasegmental   prosodic component of speech; acoustic changes across segmental level.

Sylvian fissure (sulcus)   The fissure that divides the brain into the temporal and frontal lobes. An important anatomical landmark, it runs horizontally.

taxonomic principle   learning strategy in first language development; child is limited in what ways word meanings can be extended to other objects.

telegraphic stage   stage of first language development characterized by utterances composed mostly of content words (nouns, verbs, adjectives) and very few function words (prepositions, conjunctions, affixes).

temporal lobe   area of brain associated with auditory processing; site of Wernicke's area.

tense   phonetic feature reflecting the state of the tongue muscles during vowel production.

thyroarytenoid muscle   tensing muscle of the vocal folds; also called the vocalis.

thyroid cartilage   shield-shaped cartilage composing part of the laryngeal structure; site of vocal fold and various muscle attachment.

trachea   windpipe.

tone language   language with phonemic stress levels; pitch level of a syllable influences meaning of word.

two-word stage   stage of first language development where utterances consist of two words in a syntactic and semantic relationship.

tympanic membrane   eardrum.

ultrasound   procedure, similar to sonograpy, using sound waves to observe vocal tract structures and their changes during articulation.

universal grammar   proposed set of language rules that all children are prepared to acquire in first language acquisition.

unrestricted universal   universal whose existence is independent of other occurrences in the language.

velum   soft palate; part of the vocal tract and a place of articulation.

vocal folds   source of speech sounds; two folds of tissues, muscles, and tendons that vibrate during speech production.

vocal process   section of the arytenoid cartilage where the vocal folds attach.

vocal tract   all anatomy above the vocal folds involved in speech production.

vocalis   muscles running along the length of the vocal folds; used to tense folds; also called the thyroarytenoid muscle.

voice onset time (VOT) time between the release of a stop consonant and the start of phonation; longer VOT values are associated with English voiceless stops while shorter VOT values are associated with English voiced stops.

voicing phonetic feature describing whether vocal fold vibration is present or absent during speech production.

vowel manner of speech sound with the least vocal tract obstruction of all speech sounds.

waveform visual representation of speech displaying amplitude by time.

Wernicke's aphasia syndrome of language impairment associated with damage to Wernicke's area in the left temporal lobe; characterized by fluent but nonsensical speech and impaired comprehension.

whole object principle learning strategy in first language development whereby the child assumes a label refers to the entirety of an object instead of an isolated part.

INDEX